Low Carb

The Low Carb Guide for Long-Term & Rapid Weight Loss with Nutritious Healthy Recipes

(Complete Healthy Keto Diet Delicious Recipes Cookbook)

Norman Wheeler

Published by Jason Thawne Publishing House

© Norman Wheeler

Low Carb: The Low Carb Guide For Long-term & Rapid Weight Loss With Nutritious Healthy Recipes (Complete Healthy Keto Diet Delicious Recipes Cookbook)

All Rights Reserved

ISBN 978-1-989749-44-9

This document is geared towards providing exact and reliable information in regards to the topic and issue covered. The publication is sold with the idea that the publisher isn't required to render accounting, officially permitted, or otherwise, qualified services. If advice is necessary, legal or even professional, a practiced individual in the profession should be ordered.

- From a Declaration of Principles which was accepted and approved equally by a Committee of the American Bar Association and a Committee of Publishers and Associations.

In no way is it legal to reproduce, duplicate, or even transmit any part of this document in either electronic means or in printed format. Recording of this publication is strictly prohibited and any storage of this document isn't allowed unless with proper written permission from the publisher. All rights reserved.

The information provided herein is stated to be truthful and consistent, in that any liability, in terms of inattention or otherwise, by any usage or abuse of any policies, processes, or directions contained within is the solitary and also utter responsibility of the recipient reader. Under no circumstances will any legal responsibility or blame be held against the publisher for any reparation, damages, or monetary loss due to the information herein, either directly or indirectly.

Respective authors own all copyrights not held by the publisher.

The information herein is offered for just informational purposes solely, and is universal as so. The presentation of the information is without contract or any type of guarantee assurance.

The trademarks that are used are without any consent, and also the publication of the trademark is without permission or backing by the trademark owner. All trademarks and brands within this book are for clarifying purposes only and are the owned by the owners themselves, not affiliated with this document.

TABLE OF CONTENTS

PART 1 1

INTRODUCTION 1

CHAPTER 1 – RATIONALE OF THE "EATING FATS & LOSING WEIGHT" REGIMEN 5

CHAPTER 2 – REGIMEN REALIZATION 14

RUNNING THE REGIMEN 15
REGIMEN'S REFERENCES 16

CHAPTER 3 – ROSTER OF REGULATED RATIONS 18

RECOMMENDED REGULATED RATIONS 18
SPICES 25
SWEETENERS 26
VEGETABLES 26
RESTRICTED RATIONS 28

CHAPTER 4 – GROCERY GUIDE 31

CONDIMENTS 31
COOKING OR BAKING INGREDIENTS 32
DAIRY PRODUCTS 33
DELI MEATS 34
FRUITS 34
LOW-CARBOHYDRATE VEGETABLES 35
MEATS AND POULTRY 36
NUTS AND SEEDS 36
PANTRY 36

SEAFOOD	37
MISCELLANEOUS	38
CHAPTER 5 – REGIMEN RECIPES	**39**
BREAKFAST RECIPES	39
SAUSAGE AND SPINACH FRITTATA	*39*
CREAM CHEESE PANCAKES	*41*
APPLE & ALMOND BUTTER CEREAL	*44*
DESSERTS & SWEETS RECIPES	45
CHOCOLATE DELIGHT	*45*
DAIRY-FREE, SOY-FREE VANILLA PUDDING	*47*
IRISH POTATO CANDY	*49*
COCONUT CANDY	*50*
ENTRÉE RECIPES	51
CHEESY CAULIFLOWER GRATIN	*51*
CHEESY CHILI SPAGHETTI SQUASH CASSEROLE	*53*
SUN-DRIED TOMATO & FETA MEATBALLS	*55*
CUBAN POT ROAST RECIPE	*57*
SALAD RECIPES	59
BROCCOLI SLAW	*59*
EASY LOW-CARB EGG SALAD	*61*
ANTI PASTA CAULIFLOWER SALAD	*62*
CHIA BALSAMIC DRESSING	*64*
SOUP RECIPES	65
CHICKEN VEGETABLE SOUP	*65*
CHICKEN AND CABBAGE PUREE	*67*
NO-MATZO BALL SOUP	*68*
SPINACH AND ARTICHOKE SOUP	*70*
CHAPTER 6 – 7-DAY MEAL PLAN	**73**
DAY 1 LCHF MEAL PLAN	74

DAY 2 LCHF MEAL PLAN 75
DAY 3 LCHF MEAL PLAN 77
DAY 4 LCHF MEAL PLAN 78
DAY 5 LCHF MEAL PLAN 79
DAY 6 LCHF MEAL PLAN 80
DAY 7 LCHF MEAL PLAN 82

CHAPTER 7 – REGIMEN RENDERINGS 83

WEIGHT LOSS 83
APPETITE SUPPRESSION 84
BRAIN DISORDER TREATMENT 84
DESTROY ABDOMINAL FATS 85
INCREASE HDL (GOOD) CHOLESTEROL LEVELS 86
LOWER INSULIN AND BLOOD SUGAR LEVELS 87
METABOLIC SYNDROME THERAPY 87
REDUCE LDL (BAD) CHOLESTEROL LEVELS 88
DECREASE HIGH BLOOD PRESSURE 88
REDUCE TRIGLYCERIDES 89
MISCELLANEOUS POSSIBLE APPLICATIONS 89

CHAPTER 8 – PROGRAM'S PRACTICE POINTERS 92

TIPS AND TECHNIQUES 92
DINING-OUT DO'S & DON'TS 97

CONCLUSION 101

PART 2 105

CHAPTER ONE 106

WHAT TO EAT FOR BREAKFAST WHILE TRYING TO LOSE WEIGHT 106

CHAPTER TWO 117

DIFFERENT TYPES OF FOOD FOR LUNCH TO HELP YOU LOSE WEIGHT 117

CHAPTER THREE... 125

A LIST OF SNACKS WHILE TRYING TO LOSE WEIGHT........ 125

CHAPTER FOUR.. 132

DIFFERENT TYPES OF FOOD TO EAT FOR DINNER WHILE ON A DIET.. 132

WEIGHT LOSS JOURNEY CONCLUSION............................. 141

CONCLUSION 144

ABOUT THE AUTHOR... 144

Part 1

Introduction

Low-carbohydrate and high fat (LCHF) diets have been around for such a long time, yet oftentimes disputed. Fat-conscious medical practitioners have primarily condemned their principles and methodologies. The media even joined the disapprobation bandwagon by sensationalizing to suppress completely the controversy to all. Both sectors professed that such certain diets increase the body's cholesterol levels and result to heart ailments, obviously due to the high fat content these diets entail.

However, with the changing times, there have been so many persistent dietary studies conducted about low-carbohydrate and high fat regimens. More often than not, LCHF diets were conclusively the most favorable compared against and among the popular and specific diets.

The LCHF diet does not only manifest increased body weight loss, but it also indicates principal improvements in most health risk factors, which include cholesterol levels. With the several proven health benefits it continuously provides, the LCHF diet has evolved into several modifications. Among the most accepted adaptations is the ketogenic diet.

The ketogenic diet is an exclusively high-fat eating regimen, popularly practiced for the more complicated treatments of seizures. Nevertheless, nobody really knows about the working mechanisms of the ketogenic diet, especially, on controlling seizures. Although there have been so many theories and hypotheses about how it works, the only certainty upon practicing it is the occurrence of metabolic changes that influences the chemistry of the brain.

Vegetable oils, heavy cream, and butter, commonly provide the necessary fats while at the same time, eliminating fully the sweets. While other carbohydrate-rich foods have no room in the LCHF diet's strictest essence, the regimen actually tolerates their inclusion on more generous ways.

The following pages direct you towards learning upon the rationale and working mechanisms of the LCHF diet. While it may have similar references with the ketogenic diet of achieving an ideal metabolic state of ketosis, this eBook speaks about the regimen as an established medical nutrition therapy of eating fats in order to lose weight.

Furthermore, your awareness will set you up realizing or implementing properly the LCHF regimen, including making logical decisions upon choosing the ideal food for you from among the recommended food list, as well as refraining from consuming certain restricted foods. With a concrete shopping list, you may now create your own LCHF recipes, as presented by some inspiring, easy to do, yet, delectable samples herein.

You will further be motivated upon learning important tips and techniques to help you succeed on your desire to lose weight thru indulging the LCHF diet. Indeed, the regimen not only provides you with a clear path towards shedding extra poundage, but also offers you with several health benefits.

Lead your way towards the safer habits and fondness of eating fat in order to lose weight, and onwards to good health, body comfort and total happiness! Read on to fruition… to proper nutrition… to wellness… to weighing less!

Chapter 1 – Rationale of the "Eating Fats & Losing Weight" Regimen

Foremost, this opening chapter will help you to attain a better and deeper understanding and knowledge about the LCHF diet; and, why most medical experts and health practitioners believe it is very beneficial for your weight-loss program and general body wellness, especially in the chemistry of your brain.

Roots of the Regimen

For the past thousands of years, fasting, low-carbohydrate and other similar regimen related to the LCHF diets became a common practice to treat conditions like epilepsy. Jumping on the timeline to modern times in 1921, Dr. Rawle Geyelin presented a report to the American Medical Association, where he declared the notable beneficial results of several children after undergoing fasting. All his patients have recorded lesser seizures and other epileptic attacks, and the effects had all seemed to be enduring.

Geyelin's further research and studies continued until he developed a more acceptable low-carbohydrate and high-fat diet. The succeeding years have found physicians applying the diet to their epileptic patients. However, the practice had seen a drastic decline with the advent and introduction of modern anti-epileptic medications, coupled by its sensationalized reputation as a starvation regimen.

Despite the fact that the LCHF diet was developed primarily for the treatment of epilepsy, the diet had sparked a renewed interest during the recent past as more and more people have recognized several medical and scientific studies that have shown proofs about the diet's numerous health and therapeutic benefits aside from the treatment of epilepsy. Current research, however, continues trying to unveil its mysteries thru experiments on laboratory specimens.

State of Ketosis: The Working Principle of the Regimen

Essentially, the working mechanism of the "Eating Fats & Losing Weight" regimen is to allow our bodies to enter a metabolic state known as ketosis through low-protein, low-carb, and high-fat consumptions. Ketosis is the abnormal process of manifesting an increase or accumulation of ketones. Ketones are acidic chemical molecules in the blood stream, such as blood sugar, produced by the liver's breaking down of body fats for energy. They become energy for our muscles and organs, and even for our brains.

Our bodies fundamentally use and depend upon the energy obtained from glucose, produced from our normal-to-high carbohydrate consumptions. However, when there are restricted supplies of glucose — limited carbohydrates — our metabolism shifts into a fat utilization process, wherein the liver begins producing ketones.

To enhance the production of ketone bodies, there should be reduced quantities of insulin in the bloodstream. Lower insulin levels mean sufficiently large amounts of ketone production, which is relatively the maximum effect when taking a low-carbohydrate diet.

This metabolic condition — ketosis— may appear in various forms, such as starvation, alcoholism and Type 1 diabetes mellitus. It is a state when the body's fat-burning rate is extremely high. Ketones in our blood begin to rise during this state.

Ketones may increase blood acidity that leads to some critical conditions, and thus, it is obvious that starvation is an ill-advised notion. When left unchecked, ketosis may affect urine, and result to serious kidney and liver failure.

Therefore, when planning to start implementing the regimen, close supervision from your medical adviser is highly necessary. When performed properly and responsibly, the LCHF diet can be an effective treatment for several health problems.

Attainment of Optimal Ketosis

Many practitioners of a strict low-carb regimen are often surprised to find out that their blood ketone levels are way beyond the ideal numbers. Whys is this so?

The formula is not only avoiding all carbohydrate-derived foods, but also being cautious with the intake of protein. Eating large amounts of protein allows the body to convert the excess proteins into glucose. Besides, a massive protein intake may increase insulin levels that compromise the occurrence of optimal ketosis.

As a resolve, it is usually advisable to satisfy eating with more fats. Odd as it may seem, it creates wonders though. For instance, when having a bigger serving of butter on a steak, the chances or even thoughts of taking another helping of steak diminish, if not, quashed. Instead, you will fully have your fill after having the first serving of steak.

Another popular example of a formulaic style of ingesting more fats that is worth mentioning is taking the noted Magic Bullet Coffee (MBC) or fat coffee, where the brew uses a tablespoon each of coconut oil and butter, and blended for the proper texture.

In principle, the intake of more fats enables you to be more full, and thereby, ensuring lesser protein and carbohydrate intakes. Insulin levels will surely drop, and eventually, the body achieves optimal ketosis. More importantly, fat consumption addresses directly overweight issues.

To experience the optimum hormonal effects from taking a low-carb regimen is being under the state of optimal ketosis for a prolonged duration. Under the condition of ketosis, and there is no occurrence of a reduction in weight, it is then certain that many carbohydrates are excluded in the weight issue, and are not the problems to weight loss. Note that there are other causes for obesity, and of being overweight.

Measurements of Ketones

Measuring ketones in urine samples is using the traditional spot test of using dipsticks, purchased from pharmacies. A dipstick, usually chemically coated, changes its color as it reacts with the presence of ketone bodies when dipped in a urine sample. However, there are now relatively priced gadgets to measure ketone levels, though they require a prick of a needle on a finger. Within seconds, blood ketone levels are already determined.

It is ideal to measure ketones with an empty stomach, preferably before breakfast. The presence of ketone bodies in the urine signifies the body's utilization of fat for energy instead of glucose, since insulin is not sufficiently available of using glucose to convert it into energy.

The following are the guidelines in interpreting various results of measurement values:

Lesser than 0.5 mmol/L – indicates a level, which is way beyond optimum fat burning, and it is not considered as in a state of ketosis.

Within 0.5-1.5 mmol/L – signifies receiving better effects in weight, but not in optimum conditions, and considered under light nutritional ketosis.

Around 1.5 – 3 mmol/L – are recommended levels for maximum weight reduction, and is the ideal state of reaching optimum ketosis.

Greater than 3 mmol/L – are negligible values since they denote achieving neither better nor worse outcomes than levels around 1.5-3 mmol/L. Sometimes, greater values may also connote that the body is not consuming enough food.

It is noteworthy that although ketosis usually relates to fasting or starvation, you should not confuse the LCHF diet as a form of intermittent fasting, which is completely another different type or discipline of dieting.

Cautionary Measures about the Regimen

When you have acquired Type 1 diabetes mellitus, you should never follow the advice of achieving optimal ketosis as it may pose further harm on your health. However, if ketones are indeed present in your blood, ensure that your blood sugar must be at normal levels. A normal blood sugar level is under normal ketosis, just as the ketosis possessed by healthy individuals who practice a strict low-carb regimen.

On the other hand, a high blood sugar level with high blood ketones demonstrates that insulin levels are pathologically low. Although non-diabetics do not actually suffer from these risky levels, this condition may result to ketoacidosis or diabetes acidosis, which is a possible life-threatening situation.

When this occurs, the body requires more injections of insulin in the body. Nevertheless, it is always better to consult a medical expert when you are never certain at all. Coveting high blood ketones for weight control is never worth the risk for Type 1 diabetics.

Chapter 2 – Regimen Realization

The LCHF diet is a medical nutrition therapy, crucially involving participants from differing disciplines. The team participants may include a registered dietitian coordinating with the diet's regular program; a registered nurse familiar with the cause and effects of the diet; and, a neurologist experienced in prescribing the LCHF diet.

Further assistance may be availing the services of a certified medical social practitioner working with the family, and a registered pharmacist advising upon the carbohydrate values and content of prescribed medicines. Finally, for its safe implementation, immediate members of the family and other caregivers must have the necessary knowledge about the several aspects of the diet.

Implementing the LCHF diet may pose difficulties for caregivers, as well as to the patient or practitioner due largely to the time devoted and spent regarding the planning and measuring of meals. As it is always the case, any meal unplanned may possibly break the momentum of the regular requirements of nutritional balance.

However, just as achieving success in every discipline, one requires determination and discipline. Besides, just as any aspect in educating, training, and implementing, the difficulties are always only at the beginning. On hindsight, it is just simply reciting your ABC and counting 123!

Running the Regimen

When planning to implement the LCHF diet, heed the cautionary advices of availing the necessary close supervision from your medical adviser on the diet due to the risk of complications during the regimen's initiation. For instance, when you have acquired Type-1 diabetes mellitus, do not heed the aforementioned advice on optimal ketosis, as it may pose further harm on your health. Nevertheless, if ketones are indeed present in your blood, ensure your blood sugar must be at normal levels.

A normal blood sugar level is at normal ketosis, just as the ketosis possessed by healthy individuals who practice a strict low-carb regimen. On the other hand, a high blood sugar level with high blood ketones demonstrates that insulin levels are pathologically low.

Although non-diabetics do not suffer actually from these risky levels, this condition may result to ketoacidosis, or diabetes acidosis, which is a possible life-threatening situation. As this occurs, the body requires more insulin injections. However, prudence always dictates consulting a medical expert when you are never sure at all. Coveting high blood ketones for weight control is not worth the risk for Type-1 diabetics.

Regimen's References

As the regimen takes many forms, it typically consists of daily carbohydrate restrictions not exceeding 50 grams. Foods should relatively derive their sources from vegetables, dairy, nuts, etc. Avoid refined carbohydrates and refined sugars. Thus, food must contain mostly healthy fats and protein.

Ideally, the rule of thumb to follow is the 60-35-5 formula, where 60% of calories come from fat, 35% from protein, and 5% from carbohydrates. Protein must be set at 1.5g to 1.75g for every kilogram of your ideal body weight. As a comparison, a common Western regimen comprises about 65-85% of carbohydrates, 10-20 % fat, and 5-15% protein.

Nonetheless, meals must be meticulously prepared, and accordingly measured on a weighing gram scale. Whereas, the traditional low-carb diet comprises of ratios (in grams) of protein and carbohydrates (fat to non-fat) of 3:1 and 4:1, the LCHF diet commonly consists ratios of 1:1 and 2:1.

For the regimen to be most effective, it requires the consumption of every food in its entirety. It is also noteworthy to regulate proteins, since high-protein consumptions prevent your body from undergoing optimal ketosis.

Chapter 3 – Roster of Regulated Rations

Undergoing any diet is never the easiest thing to perform in the world, especially when you are gullible and unaware about what you ought to consume or eat. This chapter lays out together the selected LCHF diet food list to help you make prudent decisions on what you should be eating and/or shopping.

Recommended Regulated Rations

Beverages

Dehydration is a common occurrence when undergoing the LCHF diet since the regimen produces a natural diuretic effect. So, whether or not you are prone to bladder pains or have urinary tract infections, you must be prepared to take plenty of liquids to keep hydrated. However, be careful with liquids using sweeteners as they can contain carbohydrates.

Carbohydrates

What chiefly determines a diet as LCHF is the value of the consumption of carbohydrates, including a person's own body metabolism and level of activity. Generally, a diet is considerably LCHF when it has a daily composition of less than 50 or 60 grams of net or effective carbohydrates.

However, individuals with healthy metabolisms are able to consume more than 100 grams of net carbohydrates daily, yet, retain good levels of ketosis, while older people with Type-2 diabetes mellitus may have to consume less than 30 grams net to obtain similar levels.

Dairy Products

As much as possible, dairy sources of a LCHF diet are preferably raw and organic.

Qty.	LCHF Diet Dairy Source	Calories	Net Carbs grams	Protein grams
8 oz.	Buttermilk, low-fat	98	12.0	8.0
1 oz.	Cheese, Blue	100	0.7	6.0
1 oz.	Cheese, Brie	95	0.1	5.9
1 oz.	Cheese, Cheddar	114	0.4	7.0
1 oz.	Cheese, Colby	112	0.7	6.7
1 oz.	Cheese, Cottage, 2%	24	1.0	3.4
1 oz.	Cheese, Cream, block	97	1.2	1.7
1 oz.	Cheese, Feta,	75	1.2	4.0
1 oz.	Cheese, Gjetost	132	12.0	2.7
1 oz.	Cheese, Monterey Jack	106	0.2	6.9
1 oz.	Cheese, Mozzarella	85	0.6	6.3
1 oz.	Cheese, Parmesan, hard	111	0.9	10.0
1 oz.	Cheese, Swiss	108	1.5	7.6
2 Tbsp.	Cream, half-n-half	39	1.2	0.9
2 Tbsp.	Cream, heavy	104	0.8	0.6
2 Tbsp.	Cream, Sour, full fat	46	0.7	0.5
2 Tbsp.	Cream, light whipping	88	0.9	0.7
1 oz.	Crème Fraiche	103	0.9	0.7
1 oz.	String cheese snack	80	1.0	6.0
8 oz.	Milk, whole	149	11.7	7.7
8 oz.	Milk, 2%	122	11.7	8.0
8 oz.	Milk, skim	83	12.2	8.3
8 oz.	Eggnog, full fat	224	20.5	11.6

Fats and Oils

Fats will be the major source of a daily calorie intake under a LCHF diet. Hence, choices shall conform to the digestion system in mind.

While fats are essential to our bodies, they may also pose as risks when we consume the wrong types of fats. Saturated and monounsaturated fats are chemically stable like, avocado, butter, coconut oil, egg yolks, and macadamia nuts. Such fats are more preferred since they are less inflammatory to most people.

Shy away from hydrogenated lards, like margarine, in order to minimize trans-unsaturated fat consumption. Besides, studies have linked these fats to higher risks of heart disease. When using vegetable oils like, flax, olive, safflower or soybean, select the cold- pressed types whenever available.

Thus, always opt for non-hydrogenated fats like, ghee liquid butter, beef tallow, or coconut oil. These fats have higher smoke points than other oils and allow lesser oxidization, thereby, providing more essential fatty acids.

Your meals may combine oils and fats into many different ways; either in dressings or sauces, or simply topping butter on cooked meat. Just be cautious about consuming nut or seed-based oils – almond oil, flaxseed oil, sesame oil, and any nuts other than macadamia and walnuts – since they are positively high in inflammatory Omega-6.

Nuts and Seeds

Nuts and seeds are excellent in a LCHF diet, especially when roasted to remove anti-nutrient components. They are, however, high in Omega-6 fatty acids. Almonds, macadamias, pecans, and walnuts are ideal in terms of carbohydrate values.

Nut and seed flours like milled flax seed and almond flour, can be great alternatives for regular flour. While the LCHF diet prohibits nothing about nuts, a proper intake balance and careful monitoring is necessary for the consumption of nuts with higher carbohydrate counts, such as pistachios, chestnuts, and cashews.

LCHF Diet Nuts and Seeds Sources dry-roasted (1 ounce)	Calories	Net Carb gram	Protein gram
Almonds	161	2.9	6.0
Brazil Nuts	184	1.3	4.0
Cashews	155	8.4	4.3
Chestnuts, European	60	13.6	0.9
Chia Seeds	139	1.7	4.0
Coconut, dried and unsweetened	185	2.0	2.0
Flax Seeds	150	0.5	5.0
Hazelnuts	176	2.3	4.0
Macadamia Nuts	201	1.5	2.0
Peanuts	166	3.8	6.7
Pecans	193	1.1	2.7
Pine Nuts	188	2.7	3.8
Pistachios	156	5.8	6.0
Pumpkin Seeds	163	2.2	8.5
Sacha Inchi Seeds (Inca peanut)	190	2.2	9.4
Sesame Seeds	161	2.6	4.8
Sunflower Seeds	165	3.7	5.5
Walnuts	183	1.9	7.0

Protein

As you primarily reduce the carbohydrates in your diet, it does not appear as if the quantity of protein you consume is as necessary to ketosis as it often becomes eventually. For instance, individuals under the Atkins diet— another popular weight-loss system based on a high-protein, high fat, and low-carbohydrate diet— often consume large quantities of protein during the early phases and remain under the state of ketosis.

However, most people must need to be extra cautious about the quantities of protein they consume over time, since their bodies will be adaptable with protein conversion into glucose, or gluconeogenesis.

During this stage, people should test to find out whether or not too much protein is moving them away from ketosis, and make the necessary adjustments. The best selection of protein options in a LCHF diet is opting for anything organic or grass-fed poultry, livestock, and aquamarine produce. Organic produce reduces the consumption of steroid hormone and bacteria.

Qty.	LCHF Diet Protein Source	Calories	Net Carbs grams	Protein grams
6 g	Bacon, 1 medium slice	40	0.0	2
1 oz.	Beef, Sirloin Steak	77	0.0	8
1 oz.	Beef, Ground, 4% fat.	34	0.0	7.5
1 oz.	Beef, Ground, 15% fat,	80	0.0	6.1
1 oz.	Beef, Roast, baked	67	0.0	8
1 oz.	Chicken, white meat	33	0.0	7
1 oz.	Chicken, dark meat	40	0.0	7
1/50 g	Egg, large (free-ranged)	75	0.4	6.3
1/56 g	Egg, XL (free-ranged)	81	0.4	7
1/63 g	Egg, jumbo (free-ranged)	90	0.5	7.9
1 oz.	Fish, Cod	30	0.0	6.5
1 oz.	Fish, Flounder	27	0.0	5
1 oz.	Fish, Sole	27	0.0	5
1 oz.	Fish, Salmon	60	0.0	7
1 oz.	Ham, smoked	40	1.0	5.3
1.25 oz.	Hot dog, beef	148	1.8	5
1 oz.	Lamb, ground	80	0.0	4.7
1 oz.	Lamb chop	70	0.0	7
1 oz.	Pork chop	60	0.0	7
1 oz.	Pork, roast	60	0.0	7
1 oz.	Pork ribs, spareribs	116	0.0	8
1 oz.	Scallops	23	2.0	6
1 oz.	Shrimp	26	1.0	6
1 oz.	Tuna	32	0.0	6.5
1 oz.	Turkey Breast	30	1.0	7
1 oz.	Veal, roasted	45	0.0	8

Spices

This food group can be critical in LCHF diet foods. Spices contain carbohydrates, so it is wise to consider their values.

In addition, most pre-made spice mixes have sugars added in them, so it is also better to note their nutrition labels. For salts, sea salt shall be more desired than table salt, as commonly combined with powdered dextrose.

Sweeteners

It is always prudent restricting yourself from anything sweet. The restriction tends curbing your cravings. Rather opt for artificial sweeteners when you ought to have something sweet. Choose liquid sweeteners since they do not contain extra binders like dextrose and maltodextrin.

Sweetener	Net Carbs (Per 100g)	Calories (Per 100g)
Aspartame	85	352
Erythritol	5	20
Stevia	5	20
Sucralose	0	0
Xylitol	60	240

Vegetables

Vegetables are extremely important in the composition of any healthy diet. However, some vegetables have high sugar contents and do not fit nutritionally. Organically grown above ground vegetables are the best for a LCHF diet. They are dark and leafy greens, and particularly high in nutrients while low in carbohydrates.

While both organic and non-organic vegetables may have the same nutritional values and properties, organically- based vegetables are much preferred to avoid pesticide residues.

Qty.	LCHF Diet Vegetable Source	Calories	Net Carbs grams	Protein grams
½ cup	Asparagus, cooked	20	2.0	2.0
3.5 oz.	Avocado	167	1.8	2.0
½ cup	Broccoli, cooked	27	3.0	1.9
3.5 oz.	Carrots, raw	35	5.3	0.6
1 cup	Cauliflower, cooked	34	1.9	2.9
2 oz.	Celery, raw	9	0.7	0.4
1 oz.	Cucumber, raw	4	0.9	0.2
1clove/3g	Garlic	4	0.9	0.2
½ cup	Green beans, cooked	22	2.9	1.2
1 oz.	Mushrooms, button	6	0.6	0.9
½ cup	Onion, green	16	2.3	0.9
½ cup	Onion, white, raw	32	6.0	0.9
1 oz.	Pepper, sweet, green,	6	0.8	0.2
1 oz.	Pickles, dill	7	1.0	0.3
1 oz.	Romaine lettuce	5	0.3	0.3
1 oz.	Butterhead lettuce	4	0.4	0.4
1 oz.	Shallots, raw	20	4.0	0.7
½ cup	Snow peas, cooked	34	3.4	2.6
5 oz	Spinach, raw	33	2.0	4.0
1 cup	Squash, acorn	115	21.0	2.3
1 cup	Squash, butternut	82	15.0	1.8
1 cup	Squash, summer	41	4.8	1.8
1 cup	Squash, spaghetti	42	8.0	1.0
1 oz.	Tomato, raw	5	0.7	0.2

Restricted Rations

It has always been inevitable to include inconspicuously or carelessly some foods into the LCHF diets, for as long as such inclusive foods possess notably low-carbohydrate and high fat contents. Many people think that they valuably contribute towards the diet's requirements and that should not always be the case. Therefore, hereunder is a list of foods that you must be careful:

<u>Diet Soda</u> – The LCHF diet does not really prohibit drinking diet soda since liquids are required for their hydrating purposes. Just be wary with the quantities you drink and bigger intakes of artificial sweeteners from sodas.

<u>Fruits</u> – Due to their high sugar contents (fructose), LCHF diets exclude fruits. However, their consumption is still possible for as long as following regulated portioning intakes.

<u>Medicine</u> – Certain medications, either generic or branded over the counter drugs, like cough syrups, colds and flu medicines, generally contain carbohydrates in large amounts. Beware of these medications, as there are available low-sugar and sugar-free alternative drugs.

Peppers – Incredible as it may seem, these little pungent and hot condiments contain sugars. So, watch out for them in stir-fried and chili-based food preparations. Choose green peppers instead, since the yellow and red varieties contain higher carbohydrate values.

Spices - As earlier mentioned, spices contain carbohydrates. However, there are particular spices that contain more carbohydrates than others do, such as allspice, bay leaves, cardamom, cinnamon, garlic powder, ginger, and onion powder.

Tomato-based Products – Known to be healthful, tomatoes are loaded with sugar when processed to be packaged or canned, like tomato sauces and diced tomatoes. Thus, be aware on your required portion sizes on their nutritional value labels. Sometimes, food companies are crafty to mislead nutritional values of serving sizes to make their products appear healthier.

Chapter 4 – Grocery Guide

When getting started on a LCHF diet and you are unsure of where to take off concerning about what to take, the following shopping list below comprise the most noted low-carbohydrate and high-fat foods. The low-carbohydrate list, outlined under major food groups, is by no means extensive. Yet, it directs you towards the right path and staying on course.

It is a prudent advice to better stick to consuming mostly real and fresh foods. Real foods mean unprocessed, organic, and natural foods. While canned or processed may be beneficial in a pinch, especially when you want to take anything quick with low carbohydrate contents, it is always much healthier taking foods in their most natural form.

Condiments

- Capers
- Cider and wine vinegars (use balsamic vinegar sparingly)

- Horseradish
- Lemon or lime juice (1 gram of carb per tablespoon)
- Mayonnaise (seek brands with the lowest carbohydrate contents)
- Most bottled hot sauces (like sriracha, sambal oelek, Tabasco)
- Most salsas
- Mustard (except sweetened mustards like, honey mustard)
- Olives
- Sugar-free dill pickles or relish: use for tuna or egg salad
- Sugar-free salad dressings
- Tamari soy sauce (when gluten sensitive, avoid soy sauce)

Cooking or Baking Ingredients

- Almond flour or other nut flours and flour substitutes; store in freezer
- Broth or bouillon

- Cocoa powder (unsweetened)
- Erythritol, Xylitol and other sugar alcohol sweeteners
- Extracts (vanilla, lemon, almond, etc.) – avoid the ones with sugar.
- Extra-virgin olive oil
- Gelatin (plain)
- Herbs and spices (ensure to be sugar-free)
- Peanut oil and coconut oil for cooking
- Sesame oil for salad dressings
- Splenda® or other artificial sweeteners like Swerve®
- Whey protein powder, plain, vanilla and chocolate flavors
- Xanthan gum for thickening and binding

Dairy Products

- Butter

- Cheese (hard) like parmesan and cheddar
- Cheese (soft) like farmer's and Muenster
- Cream cheese
- Eggs
- Full-fat or plain Greek yogurts, with carbohydrate counts of not more than seven per serving
- Heavy cream
- Sour cream

Deli Meats

- Bologna and Salami
- Cold cuts, like pastrami and turkey breast
- Pepperoni slices or sticks
- Prosciuttos

Fruits

- Avocados: great snack with lemon juice or balsamic, or make guacamole for dipping low-carb veggies
- Eat fresh fruit with a fat such as, peanut butter, whipped cream, or cheese. It slows down spikes of blood sugar.
- Fruits are optional and depend upon a stabilized health and weight. While some people cannot handle fructose, others can and remain slim and healthy. When indulging with fruits, opt for fresh local fruits in season, and prefer sticking to typically low-sugar content fruits like, berries.

Low-Carbohydrate Vegetables

- Bell peppers
- Broccoli
- Cabbage
- Cauliflower
- Cucumbers
- Leafy green vegetables, as kale and spinach

- Lettuce
- Onions and garlic
- Sprouts, Brussels or kale
- Summer squash, as zucchini

Meats and Poultry

- Bacon, ham and sausage
- Beef or pork loins, ribs, ground, chops, steaks, roasts and tips
- Chicken or Turkey, whole or parts or ground

Nuts and Seeds

- Nuts: almonds, hazelnuts, macadamias, pecans and walnuts
- Seeds: sunflower, pumpkin and sesame seeds

Pantry

- Bottled/packed low-carbohydrate vegetables: green beans, greens, okra, and sauerkraut, with no added sugars

- Broth/Stock: chicken or vegetable
- Canned anchovies, crab, salmon, sardines, shrimp, and tuna
- Canned processed meats: luncheon meat, Vienna sausage
- Canned vegetables: artichoke hearts, chipotle peppers, green chilies, hearts of palm, mushrooms, roasted red peppers, and sun-dried tomatoes in oil
- Nut butters: natural or unsweetened (keep refrigerated upon opening)
- Sauces: Alfredo, pasta, and pizza, with no added sugars or thickeners
- Tomato products: canned tomato paste and tomatoes

Seafood

- Fresh or canned salmon
- Fresh or frozen fish, scallops,
- Fresh or frozen, easy-to-peel shrimp
- Tuna in oil or water

This would include any type or kind of seafood; best options are preferably wild farmed or caught since fat levels of Omega-3 are higher.

Miscellaneous

- Beef jerky or beef sticks
- Pork rinds (crushed, a better alternative for bread crumbs)

Chapter 5 – Regimen Recipes

Breakfast Recipes

Sausage and Spinach Frittata

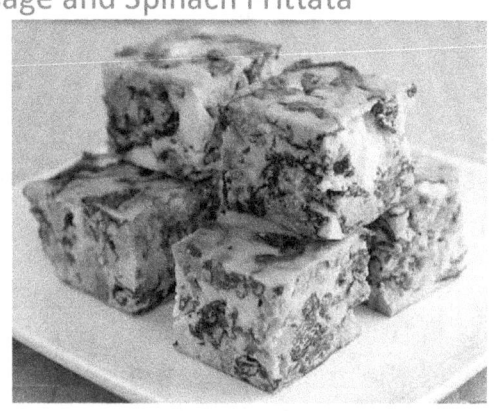

Ingredients	Yield: 12 squares
12 ounces	sausage
10 ounces	frozen chopped spinach, thawed and drained
½ cup	Feta cheese, crumbled
12 pieces	eggs
½ cup	heavy cream
½ cup	almond milk, unsweetened
½ tsp	salt
¼ tsp	black pepper

¼ tsp   ground nutmeg

Directions

1. Slice the raw sausage into small pieces, and place them in a medium-sized bowl.

2. Ensure that the spinach is squeezed-dry from any remaining liquid after washing. Break the spinach up into the same bowl as the sausage.

3. Sprinkle feta cheese over the mixture. Toss lightly until fully combined. Lightly spread the mixture onto a greased 13" x 9" casserole dish.

4. In a larger bowl, combine almond milk, cream, nutmeg, salt and pepper with the beaten the eggs together, and mix until well blended.

5. Gently pour the mixture into the dish until about ¾ full.

6. Bake at 375oF for 50 minutes until fully set. Serve warm or at room temperature.

Nutritional Values per Serving: 206 calories | 16g fat | 1.4g net carbohydrates | 12g protein

Serving Size: One 3-inch square

Cream Cheese Pancakes

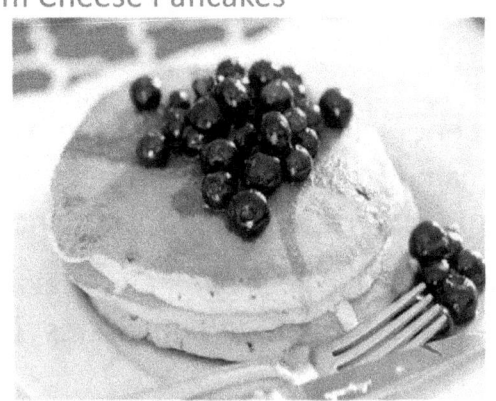

Ingredients	Yield: Four 6-inch diameter pancakes>
2 ounces	cream cheese
2 pieces	eggs
1 packet	sweetener
½ tsp	cinnamon

Directions

1. Combine all ingredients in a blender. Blend until smooth. Allow to stand for 2 minutes for the bubbles to settle.

2. Pour ¼ of the batter into a hot pan greased with butter. Cook for 2 minutes until golden. Flip and cook 1 minute on the other side.

3. Repeat the procedure with the remaining batter. Serve with sugar-free syrup and fresh berries of your choice.

<u>Nutritional values per batch:</u> 344 calories | 29g fat | 2.5g net carbohydrates | 17g protein

<u>Serving Size:</u> One 6-inch diameter pancake

Scrambled Eggs with Mayonnaise

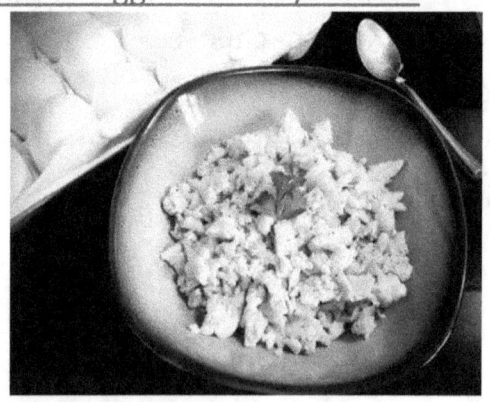

Ingredients   <u>Yield:</u> One serving

50 g raw egg
23 g mayonnaise (organic)
10 g butter

Pinch of salt to taste

Directions

1. Melt butter in asmall non-stick pan.
2. Mix the mayonnaise and egg together with a fork until fully combined.
3. Cook the egg and mayo mixture in butter. Use asilicone spatulato gently fold the egg mixture until it is set.
4. Scrape the eggs and all the remaining fat onto a serving plate and serve immediately.

<u>Nutritional values per serving:</u> 308 Calories | 31.27g fat | 0.53g net carbohydrates | 6.38g protein

<u>Serving size:</u> Entire serving

Apple & Almond Butter Cereal

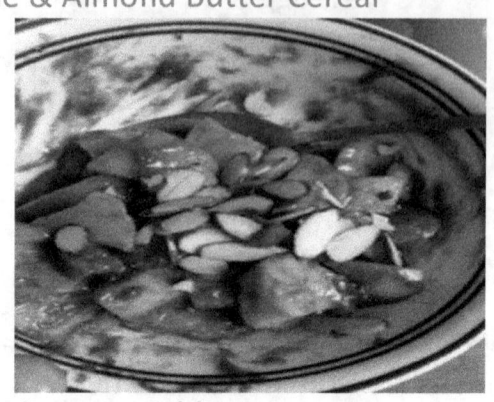

Ingredients	Yield: One serving
38 g	almond butter
30 g	apple sauce, unsweetened
9 g	coconut oil, melted
0.2 g – 1 g	ground cinnamon
2 Tbsp	almonds, sliced (optional)

Pinch of salt to taste

Directions

1. Combine all ingredients together in a small bowl.

2. Stir well until all the ingredients are evenly integrated.

3. When the mixture is too thick, thin the consistency with water. If desired, add sliced almonds.

Nutritional values per serving: 305 calories | 36.4g fat | 5.46g net carbohydrates | 8.4g protein

Serving size: Entire serving

Desserts & Sweets Recipes

Chocolate Delight

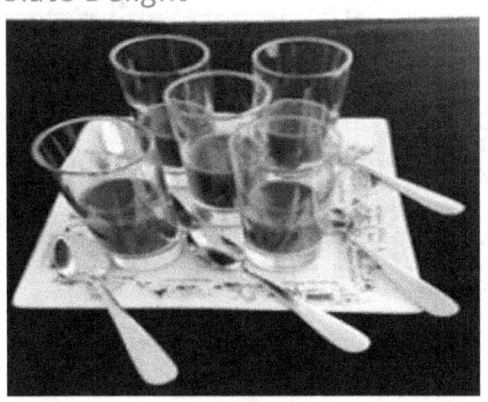

Ingredients	Yield: Five servings
3 Tbsp+2 tsp / 69 g	coconut oil
2 Tbsp+2 tsp / 40 g	medium chain triglyceride (MCT) oil
1 tsp / 5 g	sunflower seeds, ground

7 g	cocoa powder, unsweetened
2 tsp / 10 g	sugar-free syrup, chocolate
1 tsp / 5 g	sugar-free syrup, peppermint

Directions

1. Combine MCT oil and coconut oil. Stir until coconut oil melts.
2. Stir sugar-free syrups, sunflower seeds, and cocoa into oils.
3. Pour by dividing evenly into 5 small containers. Refrigerate until firm.

<u>Nutritional values per serving:</u> 200 calories | 22g fat | 0.4g net carbohydrates | 0.3 gm protein

Dairy-Free, Soy-Free Vanilla Pudding

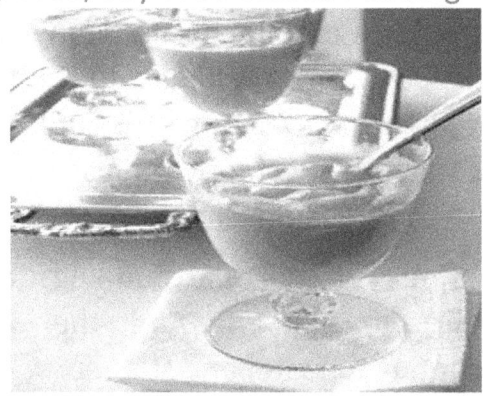

Ingredients	Yield: Two cups
400 g / 1 can	coconut milk, full fat
4 pieces / 60 g	egg yolks
4 tsp / 20 g	ghee
1/2 tsp / 2 g	pure vanilla extract
1 tsp	salt
0.1g / pinch	Xanthan gum
10 drops	Stevia liquid sweetener

Directions

1. Combine and whisk thoroughly all ingredients except the Stevia in a small saucepan.Gradually heat the mixture until it starts to steam and bubble. Stir the mixture constantly. Adjust the heat to keep a constant simmer.

2. Continue to cook the pudding until it begins to thicken. Add the Stevia according to taste, and stir very well.

3. Pour the pudding into a glass bowl, cover and refrigerate until completely chilled. Stir when ready to serve.

Nutritional values for entire recipe: 1078 calories | 107.92g fat | 12.48g net carbohydrates | 14.24g protein

Serving Size: One cup

Irish Potato Candy

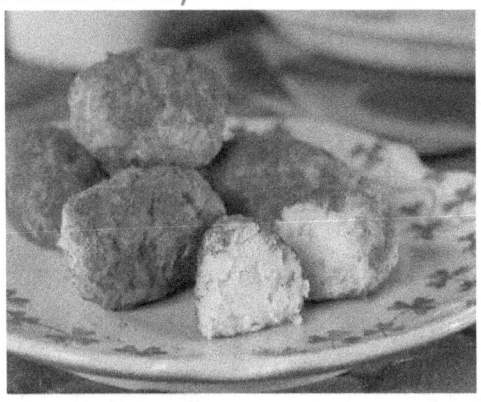

Ingredients	Yield: Eight 50-calorie servings
69 g	Philadelphia Cream Cheese
7 g	butter, at room temperature
16 g	shredded coconut, unsweetened
2 g	ground cinnamon

Sweetener of choice

Directions

1. Combine all of the ingredients except the cinnamon in a bowl. Allow the mixture to set in the refrigerator until it has hardened.

2. Divide the batter by weight by adding the total weight of ingredients less that

of the cinnamon, and dividing by number of servings desired.

3. Roll the portions into potato-like shapes and place on a sheet of parchment paper. Sprinkle the shapes with cinnamon. Store them in the refrigerator for a week.

4. <u>Nutritional values for entire batch:</u> 401 calories | 40.85g fat | 3.57g net carbohydrates | 6.45g protein

Coconut Candy

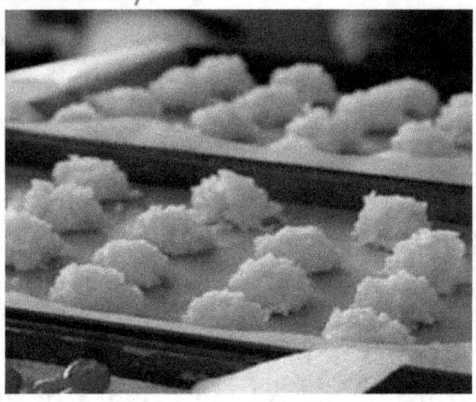

Ingredient

Coconut Butter (also known as Coconut Manna)

Directions

1. Melt the coconut butter gently just until it resembles a creamy peanut butter consistency.
2. Pour or spoon into candy molds.
3. Refrigerate for at least 10 minutes to harden. Refrigerate for up to several weeks in a closed container.

<u>Nutritional values per 15g of coconut butter:</u> 102 calories | 10.3gm fat | 1.14g net carbohydrates | 1.14g protein

Entrée Recipes

Cheesy Cauliflower Gratin

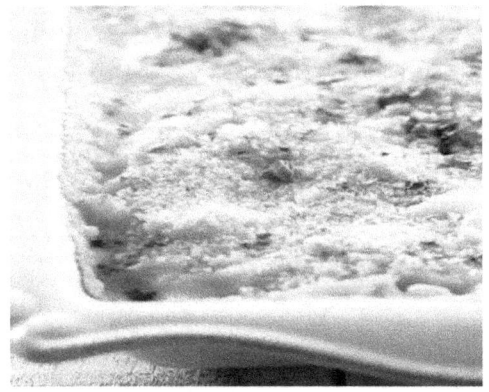

Ingredients   <u>Yield:</u> Six servings

4 cups	raw cauliflower florets
4 Tbsp	butter
⅓-cup	heavy whipping cream
6 pieces	Pepper jack cheese, deli slices

Dash of salt and pepper to taste

Directions

1. Combine all ingredients except the cheese in a microwave dish and mix thoroughly. Heat the mixture for about 25 minutes, or until tender.

2. Remove from the microwave and mash with a fork. Add more salt or pepper to taste. Lay slices of cheese over the cauliflower mixture. Heat again until the cheese melts. Serve hot.

<u>Nutritional values per serving:</u> 215 calories | 19g fat | 2g net carbohydrates | 6g protein

<u>Serving Size:</u> Approximately ¾ cup

Cheesy Chili Spaghetti Squash Casserole

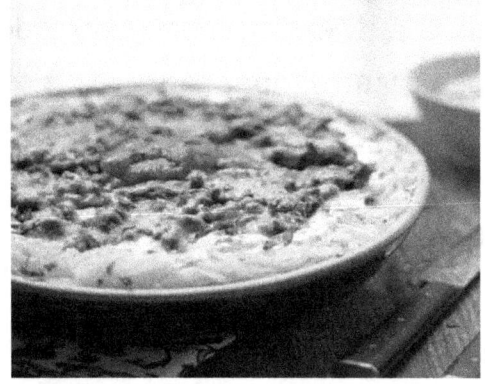

Ingredients   Yield: Eight servings

For the Chili:

1 lb	lean ground beef (or turkey)
1 tsp	ground cumin
1 tsp	ground coriander
1 Tbsp	chopped chipotles in adobo (optional)
½ tsp	garlic powder
1 tsp	dried oregano
½ cup	prepared salsa

Salt and pepper to taste

For the Casserole:

4 cups	cooked spaghetti squash
2 tbsp	butter, melted

¾ cup sour cream

1¾ cup Mexican cheese, shredded

Chopped cilantro (optional)

Sour cream, salsa, avocado to serve (optional)

Directions

For the Chili:

1. Season the ground meat with salt and pepper, and cook it in a medium-sized saucepan until browned.

2. Discard any extra fat and add the remaining the chili ingredients. Simmer for about 10 minutes.

For the Casserole:

1. Combine the cooked spaghetti squash and melted butter in a medium-sized bowl. Toss to coat the pasta with butter. Season generously with salt and pepper to taste.

2. Spread out the spaghetti squash in a 14-inch casserole dish. Sprinkle with ¾-cup of shredded cheese. Spread the sour cream over the cheese layer.

Spoon on the chili and spread it out, leaving a 1-inch border of spaghetti squash around the edge. Top with the remaining 1-cup of shredded cheese.

3. Bake at 350oF for 30 minutes. Sprinkle with cilantro and serve with sour cream, salsa, and guacamole or avocado slices as desired.

<u>Nutrition values per serving:</u> 284 calories | 20g fat | 6g net carbohydrates |23g protein

<u>Serving Size:</u> Approximately 1-½ cups

Sun-dried Tomato & Feta Meatballs

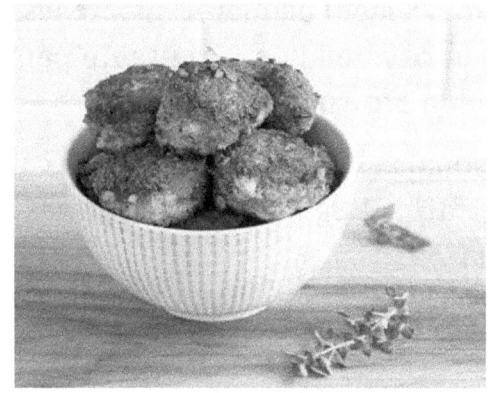

Ingredients	<u>Yield:</u> 16 meatballs
1 lb	ground turkey

¼ cup	Feta cheese, crumbled
2 Tbsp / 5 ounce	sun-dried tomatoes, chopped
1 Tbsp	fresh thyme leaves
1 piece	egg
½ tsp	garlic powder
¼ cup	almond flour
2 Tbsp	water

Olive oil for frying

Directions:

1. Combine all ingredients except olive oil in a medium bowl and mix well.
2. Form 1-inch diameter meatballs, and fry in olive oil in a large sauté pan until golden brown.

<u>Nutritional values per meatball:</u> 89 calories | 10g fat | 1.8g net carbohydrates | 6g protein

Serving Size: <u>4 meatballs</u>

Cuban Pot Roast Recipe

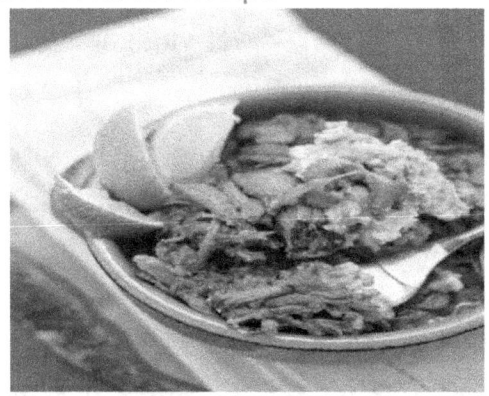

Ingredients	Yield: Ten servings
2.5-3 lb	boneless chuck roast
½ cup	Salsa Verde
½ cup	green chili, canned, chopped
1 cup	tomatoes, diced
2 Tbsp	dried onion flakes
1 tsp	garlic powder
½ cup	red and yellow peppers, cut into strips
1 tsp	salt
2 Tbsp	ground cumin
1 Tbsp	ground coriander
1 tsp	dried oregano
1 Tbsp	chili powder

½ tsp   black pepper
2 Tbsp   apple cider vinegar

Directions

1. Season the roast generously with salt and pepper. Sear in a hot pan until browned on all sides. Place the meat in the bottom of a 5-quart crock pot slow cooker.

2. In the pan where the meat was seared, add the Salsa Verde, chili, and tomatoes. Deglaze and bring to a boil.

3. Pour the mixture over the meat in the crock pot. Add all the remaining ingredients into the slow cooker and stir thoroughly.

4. Cook for 4 hours over high flame, or 6 hours over low flame, or until the meat is tender. Shred the meat and serve with toppings of your choice.

<u>Nutritional values per serving:</u> 271 calories | 19g fat | 2g net carbohydrates | 20g protein

<u>Serving Size:</u> Approximately 1 cup

Salad Recipes

Broccoli Slaw

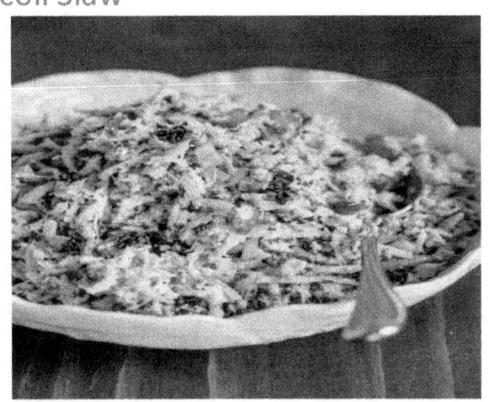

Ingredients

29 g	raw broccoli
15 g	mayonnaise
7.6 g	pomegranate seeds
7 g	macadamia nuts, crushed into small pieces
2 g	cider vinegar
1 g	Truvia sweetener

Dash of salt and pepper to taste

Directions

1. Wash the broccoli thoroughly. Cut the florets off the stem and break them into very small pieces. Shred the stems. Combine the stems and florets together until evenly incorporated. Weigh portions you just need, and then steam lightly.

2. Complete by mixing in the remaining ingredients and season to taste. It is ideal to allow sitting the recipe overnight for best results when all the flavors have ample time blending together while the broccoli has sufficient time to soften a little.

<u>Nutritional values per serving:</u> 124 calories | 10.4g fat | 9.1g net carbohydrates | 1.6g protein

Easy Low-carb Egg Salad

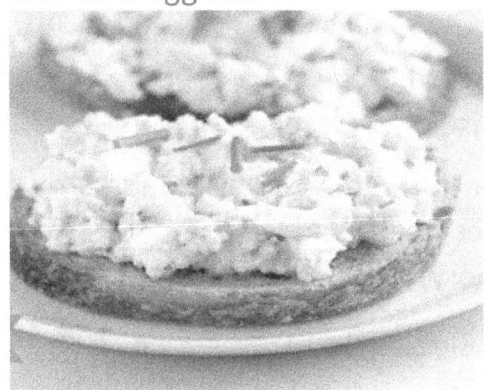

Ingredients	Yield: Four ⅓-cup servings
6 pieces	eggs
2 Tbsp	mayonnaise
1 tsp	Dijon mustard
1 tsp	lemon juice
¼ tsp	salt

Dash of kosher salt and pepper to taste

1 length celery stalk, cut into ½-inch long (optional)

Directions

1. Place the eggs gently in a medium-sized saucepan. Add cold water until the eggs are covered by about an inch. Bring to a boil for 10 minutes.

2. Remove from heat and allow cooling. Peel the eggs under running cold water. Place the eggs in a food processor and pulse until chopped.

3. Stir in the mayonnaise, mustard, lemon juice, salt and pepper. Top with cut celery, if desired.

<u>Nutritional values per serving:</u> 166 calories | 14g fat | 0.85g net carbohydrates | 10g protein

Anti Pasta Cauliflower Salad

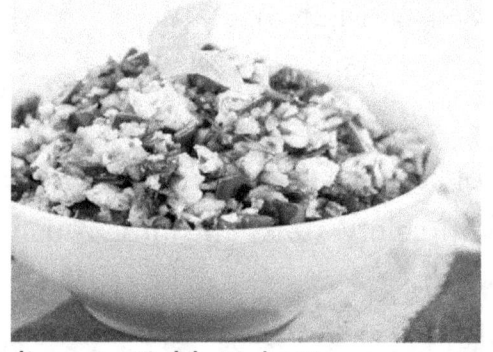

Ingredients	<u>Yield:</u> Eight ½-cup servings
2 cups	raw cauliflower, finely chopped
½ cup	radicchio, chopped

½ cup	artichoke hearts, chopped
⅓ cup	fresh basil, chopped
½ cup	Parmesan cheese, grated
3 Tbsp	sun-dried tomatoes, chopped
3 Tbsp	Kalamata olives, chopped
1 clove	garlic, minced
3 Tbsp	balsamic vinegar
3 Tbsp	extra virgin olive oil

Dash of salt and pepper to taste

Directions

1. Cook the cauliflower sans seasoning in the microwave for 5 minutes, and let it stand for cooling.
2. Combine all the dry ingredients in a medium-sized bowl. In a smaller bowl, whisk together the liquid ingredients and pour it over the salad. Toss to combine, and season with salt and pepper to taste. Serve chilled or at room temperature.

<u>Nutritional values per serving:</u> 102 calories | 8g fat | 4g net carbohydrates | 3g protein

Chia Balsamic Dressing

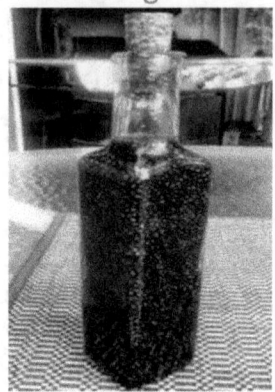

Ingredients

Yield: One serving (Serve over salad)

1tsp / 3.5 g	Chia seeds
1tsp / 5 g	white wine vinegar
1 tsp / 4 g	balsamic vinegar
1 Tbsp /14 g	olive oil

Pinch of salt to taste

Directions

1. Whisk both vinegars into the Chia seeds. Add the olive oil and whisk again.

2. Allow thedressing tosit for10 minutes as the Chia seeds absorb moisture and become plump

<u>Nutritional values per serving:</u> 140 calories | 15g fat | 1g net carbohydrates | 0.6g protein

Soup Recipes

Chicken Vegetable Soup

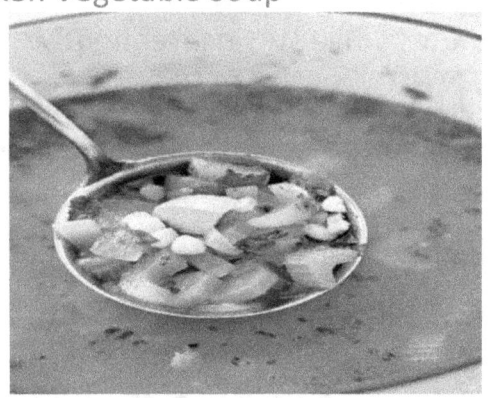

Ingredients	<u>Yield:</u> One-bowl serving
15 g	Butter, olive oil or other oils
40 g	mixed raw vegetables such as, broccoli, carrots, cauliflower, celery, green beans, onions, pepper

	spinach, and squash, finely chopped
20 g	Chicken, skinless, cooked, finely chopped
100 g	Broth, fat-free, canned

A dash of salt and pepper to taste

Directions

1. Place butter or oil in a small saucepan and heat until it starts sizzling.
2. Add the vegetables and sauté for 2 minutes while stirring frequently.
3. Add the chicken and continue sautéing to allow absorbing fat for about 1 minute.
4. Pour in the broth then stir occasionally.
5. Add a pinch of salt and pepper to taste; and if desired, add a dried herb such as basil, sage or thyme. Reduce heat and simmer for 5-10 minutes on low heat.

<u>Nutritional values per serving:</u> 168 calories | 13.4g fat | 3.2g net carbohydrates | 8.5g protein

Chicken and Cabbage Puree

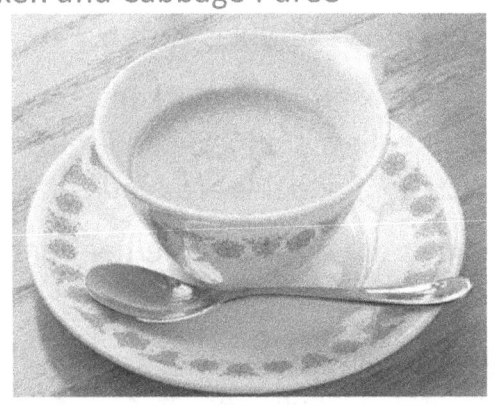

Ingredients	Yield: One-bowl serving
100 g	chicken broth
30 g	raw green cabbage, shredded
5 g	raw onion, diced small
1 g	raw garlic, diced fine
20 g	cooked chicken breast, diced
15 g	butter
15 g	olive oil
15 g	mayonnaise

Dash of salt & white pepper to taste

Directions

1. In a small pot, add olive oil and butter. Melt the butter over medium heat. Add

the cabbage, onions and garlic, and sauté until vegetables soften.

2. Add the broth and chicken. Cover the pot and allow simmering over low heat until the vegetables are tender.

3. Remove the pot from the heat and add the mayonnaise.

<u>Nutritional values per serving:</u> 397 calories | 32.5g fat | 2.5g net carbohydrates | 7.35g protein

No-Matzo Ball Soup

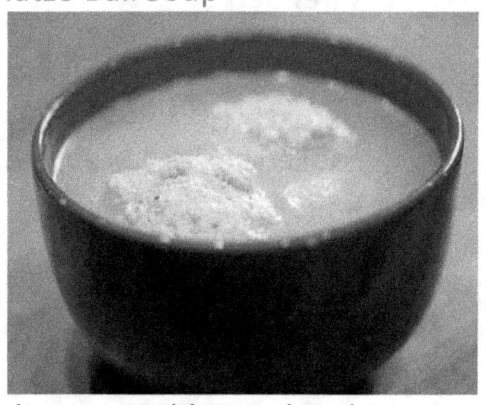

Ingredients	<u>Yield:</u> One-bowl serving
12 g	olive oil
8.5 g	coconut flour

3 g	Psyllium seed, husks or powdered
0.5 g	baking powder
0.5 g	baking soda
44 g	raw egg, mixed well
150 g	chicken broth
15 g	celery, sliced thin
10 g	raw carrots, sliced thin

Salt, pepper, garlic powder, parsley flakes, if desired

Directions

1. Combine the olive oil, coconut flour, Psyllium seed, baking powder and baking soda together in a small bowl. Stir vigorously until all of the lumps have dissolved. Add the egg and optional seasonings to the mixture. Stir vigorously again as the batter immediately thickens and become very stiff.

2. Lightly grease a microwave dish. Wet your hands with cold water and roll the batter to form 3 round balls. Place the

balls on the greased plate and heat them for 30 seconds to 1 minute.

3. Combine the broth, celery and carrots. Pour additional water when necessary. Heat the broth in the microwave until the vegetables are tender. Add the cooked matzo balls to the broth and serve immediately.

Nutritional values per serving: 206 calories | 17.59g fat | 4.2 g net carbohydrates | 7.53g protein

Spinach and Artichoke Soup

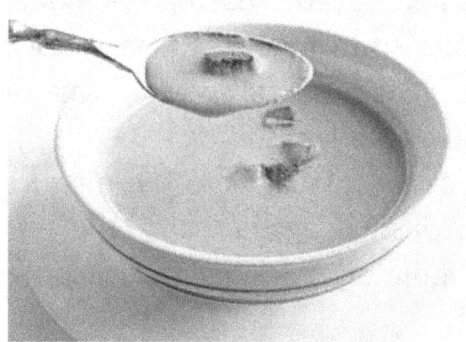

Ingredients   Yield: 4 servings
4 cups   baby spinach leaves
2 cups   canned artichoke hearts,

	drained
1 Tbsp	butter
2 slices	provolone cheese
2 oz	Dubliner or cheddar cheese
½ piece	small onion, roughly chopped
2 Tbsp	sour cream
2 cups	water
1 tsp	Sriracha hot sauce
½ cup	heavy cream
½ tsp	garlic powder

Salt and pepper to taste

Directions

1. Add all of the ingredients to a blender. Puree.

2. Pour the mixture into a medium saucepan placed over medium heat. Reduce the heat and simmer for about 15 minutes.

3. Taste to desired flavor and/or adjust by seasoning. You can add another tablespoon of butter prior to serving if you desire for a richer flavor.

<u>**Nutritional values per serving:**</u> 247 calories | 18.4g fat | 12.1 g net carbohydrates | 11.3g protein

Chapter 6 – 7-Day Meal Plan

To further facilitate planning a menu for a LCHF diet with a specific period of time, the following tables show an example of an improvised LCHF diet meal plan for a week's period.

In a detailed analysis, it can be noticed that the quantities of proteins in grams are a quite high, but in terms of the total calorie intake, the proportions of protein intake in relation to the proportions of fat intake are just ideal.

Upon having a final analysis of the meal plan, it all boils down to eating regulated servings of protein meats; adding as much fat as you like, but within calorie limits; and, opting for low-carb vegetables for each day.

Obviously, you cannot consume whole sticks of butter and expect a reduced weight. But when you are not attempting at losing weight, consuming sufficient saturated fats and adequate protein is an ideal way to suppress hunger. Hunger pangs in between meals can be capably handled through consuming high-fat, low-carb foods like, Hass avocado, or sticks of celery with almond butter, or a handful of raw almonds.

As a general rule of thumb, you can maintain a regular scope of food values, where fats are proportioned at 75%; proteins at 25%; and, carbohydrates at a maximum of 5%. When having an active lifestyle, carbohydrates can be adjusted to be increased a bit. But when undergoing a strict low-carb diet, it might be suggested for you to enforce yourself performing daily body exercises rigidly, or depending upon how your body reacts to the activity.

Day 1 LCHF Meal Plan

DAY 1	MEALS	CALORIE	FAT g	NET CARB g	PROTEIN g
BREAKFAST	3-inch square, Sausage and Spinach Frittata	206	16	1	12
	Coffee with 2-Tbsp. heavy cream	120	12	1	0
SNACK	½-Hass avocado with little salt and pepper	114	11	1	1
LUNCH	½-cup Simple Egg Salad	166	14	1	10
	4-romaine lettuce leaves	4	0	0	0
	2-slices cooked bacon	92	7	0	6
SNACK	24-raw almonds	166	5	2	6
DINNER	6-oz. rotisserie chicken	276	11	0	42
	¾-cup Cauliflower Gratin	215	19	2	6
	2-cups chopped romaine lettuce	16	0	1	1
	2-Tbsp. Caesar salad dressing (sugar-free)	170	18	2	1
DESSERT	2-squares Lindt 90% chocolate	105	9	3	3
TOTALS		*1650*	*132*	*14*	*88*

Day 2 LCHF Meal Plan

DAY 2	MEALS	CALORIE	FAT g	NET CARB g	PROTEIN g
BREAKFAST	3-inch square, Sausage and Spinach Frittata	206	16	1	12
	Coffee with 2-Tbsp. heavy cream	120	12	1	0
SNACK	5-sticks of celery with 2- Tbsp. almond butter	200	16	2.5	7
LUNCH	2-cups chopped romaine lettuce	16	0	1	1
	1-cup chopped leftover chicken	276	11	0	42
	2-Tbsp. Caesar salad dressing (sugar-free)	170	18	2	1
SNACK	½-Hass avocado with little salt and pepper	114	11	1	1
DINNER	1-Italian sausage link, cooked and sliced	230	18	1	13
	1-cup cooked broccoli	55	0	6	4
	1-Tbsp. butter	102	12	0	0
	2-Tbsp. grated Parmesan cheese	42	3	0	4
DESSERT	2-squares Lindt 90% chocolate	105	9	3	3
TOTALS		*1636*	*126*	*18.5*	*88*

Day 3 LCHF Meal Plan

DAY 3	MEALS	CALORIE	FAT g	NET CARB g	PROTEIN g
BREAKFAST	2-Cream Cheese Pancakes	172	14	1	8
	2-pcs. cooked bacon	92	7	0	6
	Coffee with 2-Tbsp. heavy cream	120	12	1	0
SNACK	2-String Cheese	160	12	2	16
LUNCH	1 Italian sausage link, cooked and sliced	230	18	1	13
	¾-cup Cauliflower Gratin	215	19	2	6
SNACK	1-cup bone broth	50	1	0	1
DINNER	1 ½-cup Chili Spaghetti Squash Casserole	284	20	6	23
	2-cups raw baby spinach	14	0	1	2
	1-Tbsp. ranch dressing (sugar-free)	70	7	1	0
DESSERT	2-squares Lindt 90% chocolate	105	9	3	3
TOTALS		*1512*	*119*	*18*	*78*

Day 4 LCHF Meal Plan

DAY 4	MEALS	CALORIE	FAT g	NET CARB g	PROTEIN g
BREAKFAST	3-inch square, Sausage and Spinach Frittata	206	16	1	12
	Coffee with 2-Tbsp. heavy cream	120	12	1	0
SNACK	½-Hass avocado with little salt and pepper	114	11	1	1
LUNCH	1 ½-cup Chili Spaghetti Squash Casserole	284	20	6	23
SNACK	1-cup bone broth	50	1	0	1
DINNER	½-cup Anti Pasta Salad	102	8	4	3
	4-Sundried Tomato and Feta Meatballs	356	32	2.5	24
	2-cups raw baby spinach	14	0	1	2
	1-Tbsp. Italian dressing (sugar-free)	35	3	0	0
DESSERT	2-squares Lindt 90% chocolate	105	9	3	3
TOTALS		*1386*	*112*	*19.5*	*69*

Day 5 LCHF Meal Plan

DAY 5	MEALS	CALORIE	FAT g	NET CARB g	PROTEIN g
BREAKFAST	2-Cream Cheese Pancakes	172	14	1	8
	2-pcs. cooked bacon	92	7	0	6
	Coffee with 2-Tbsp. heavy cream	120	12	1	0
SNACK	1-cup bone broth	50	1	0	1
LUNCH	½-cup Anti Pasta Salad	102	8	4	3
	4-Sundried Tomato and Feta Meatballs	356	32	2.5	24
SNACK	5-sticks of celery with 2-Tbsp. Almond Butter	200	16	2.5	7
DINNER	1-cup Cuban Pot Roast (taco salad style)	271	19	2	20
	2-cups chopped romaine lettuce	16	0	1	1
	2-Tbsp. sour cream	51	5	1	1
	¼-cup shredded Cheddar cheese	114	9	0.5	7
DESSERT	2-squares Lindt 90% chocolate	105	9	3	3
TOTALS		*1649*	*132*	*18.5*	*81*

Day 6 LCHF Meal Plan

DAY 6	MEALS	CALORIE	FAT g	NET CARB g	PROTEIN g
BREAKFAST	3-eggs (scrambled or fried)	215	14	1	19
	1-tsp. butter	36	4	0	0
	2-pcs. cooked bacon	92	7	0	6
	Coffee with 2-Tbsp. heavy cream	120	12	1	0
SNACK	24-raw almonds	166	15	2	6
LUNCH	1-cup Cuban Pot Roast (taco salad style)	271	19	2	20
	2-cups chopped romaine lettuce	16	0	1	1
	2-Tbsp. sour cream	51	5	1	1
	¼-cup shredded Cheddar cheese	114	9	0.5	7
SNACK	1-cup bone broth	50	1	0	1
DINNER	1 ½-cup Chili Spaghetti Squash Casserole	284	20	6	23
	2-cups raw baby spinach	14	0	1	2
	1-Tbsp. ranch dressing (sugar-free)	70	7	1	0
DESSERT	2-squares Lindt 90% chocolate	105	9	3	3
TOTALS		*1604*	*122*	*19.5*	*89*

Day 7 LCHF Meal Plan

DAY 7	MEALS	CALORIE	FAT g	NET CARB g	PROTEIN g
BREAKFAST	2-Cream Cheese Pancakes	172	14	1	8
	2-pcs. cooked bacon	92	7	0	6
	Coffee with 2-Tbsp. heavy cream	120	12	1	0
SNACK	2-String Cheese	160	12	2	16
LUNCH	4-Sundried Tomato and Feta Meatballs	356	32	2.5	24
	½-cup Anti Pasta Salad	102	8	4	3
	1-cup bone broth	50	1	0	1
SNACK	1-cup Cuban Pot Roast (taco salad style)	271	19	2	20
DINNER	2-cups chopped romaine lettuce	16	0	1	1
	2-Tbsp. sour cream	51	5	1	1
	¼-cup shredded Cheddar cheese	114	9	0.5	7
DESSERT	2-squares Lindt 90% chocolate	105	9	3	3
TOTALS		*1609*	*128*	*18*	*90*

Chapter 7 – Regimen Renderings

LCHF diets are becoming more acceptable and favored, and for a wide variety of reasons. Besides having already been established as a recommended treatment for epilepsy, and its popular effect on losing weight, LCHF diets are continuously studied by medical researchers for the prevention of other neurological and health conditions.

The following is a compilation from a June 2013 report of the European Journal of Clinical Nutrition about various health conditions that may be overcome by LCHF diets:

Weight Loss

Among the most effective and simplest ways of losing weight is cutting down on carbohydrates intake. Studies even show that individuals under a low-carb regimen tend to lose more weight much rapidly than those under low-fat diets despite the fact that the latter dieters are aggressively limiting calories.

The principal reason for this effect is that, low-carb diets impel to drain excess water from the body. Since these diets decrease the insulin levels, the kidneys begin to shed excess sodium, resulting to faster weight reduction in just a couple of weeks.

Appetite Suppression

Eating low-carbohydrate diets and more protein and fats leads to an automatic suppression of appetite, and often end up consuming much lesser calories even without trying. Obviously, a resulting reduction in weight occurs when appetite accordingly goes down.

Brain Disorder Treatment

Our brain importantly needs glucose, but only some parts of the brain burn glucose into energy. However, a greater part of the brain can also burn ketones. Ketones are created during fasting, or when there is a low consumption of carbohydrates, wherein the liver produces glucose from proteins. This is the working principle behind the LCHF diet, which has been applied for quite a long time now in the treatment of epilepsy, especially when patients are unresponsive to drug treatment.

DestroyAbdominal Fats

Fats in the body differ. Their stored location in the body determines how it affects our health. To note, the stored locations of fats are situated under the skin— subcutaneous fat; and, in the abdominal cavity— visceral fat, which tends to nestle in body organs. A high accumulation of visceral fats leads to insulin resistance, inflammation, and metabolic dysfunction.

Low-carb diets, even when compared against low-fat diets, become more effective at greatly reducing destructive abdominal fats. Moreover, a bigger percentage of those fats lost come from the abdominal cavity. With the passage of time under such a diet, the body dramatically decreases its risks to Type 2 diabetes mellitus and heart disease.

Increase HDL (Good) Cholesterol Levels

High Density Lipoprotein (HDL) and Low Density Lipoprotein (LDL) indicate the lipoproteins that transport cholesterol around the bloodstream.

While LDL bears cholesterol from the liver and towards the different parts of the body, HDL moves cholesterol away from the body and towards the liver, where it may excrete or reuse cholesterol.

Since low-carb diets tend to be high in fat, they cause impressive increases in blood levels of HDL, more popularly known as the good cholesterol. Another potential indicator of heart ailment risks is the triglycerides-HDL ratio, where a higher ratio connotes greater health risks. Low-carb diets result to enhanced ratios by lowering triglycerides while raising HDL levels.

Lower Insulin and Blood Sugar Levels

The most efficient way to lower insulin and blood sugar levels is reducing the intake of carbohydrates. In addition, a low-carb intake is a very effective way of treating, and possibly, even reversing Type-2 diabetes mellitus.

Nevertheless, when you are under current medication on lowering blood sugar levels, it is highly advised to consult with your physician prior to devising changes in your carbohydrate consumption, since your dosage may require adjustments to avoid hypoglycemia.

Metabolic Syndrome Therapy

The metabolic syndrome is a collection of the following symptoms:

Abdominal obesity,

High blood pressure,

Increased blood sugar levels,

High levels of triglycerides; and,

Low HDL levels

With a low-carb diet, it effectively alters and reverses all the aforementioned symptoms greatly related to heart disease and diabetes risks.

Reduce LDL (Bad) Cholesterol Levels

People having high levels of LDL, commonly known as the bad cholesterol, are more prone to undergo heart attacks.

However, what matters most is the type of LDL, particularly the size of its particles. Individuals having mostly smaller particles incur higher risks of heart disease, while people with mostly larger particles entail lower risks.

Studies show that low-carb diets enhance the sizes of LDL particles from small to large, and at the same time, reducing the amounts of LDL particles in the bloodstream.

Decrease High Blood Pressure

High blood pressure, or hypertension, is a major risk factor for many ailments, including stroke, heart disease, kidney failure and more. Studies have shown that reducing carbohydrate consumptions causes significant reduction in blood pressure, and thereby, reduced risks of several common diseases.

Reduce Triglycerides

Triglycerides are fat molecules in the blood, and noted risk factors for heart ailments. Low-carb diets are very effective at drastically decreasing blood triglycerides as compared to low-fat diets, where blood triglycerides tend to increase in most instances.

Miscellaneous Possible Applications

Further medical studies declare that the LCHF diet effectively treats many rare metabolic diseases. There have been case reports indicating its possible treatment for a certain type of brain tumor—astrocytomas.

In other smaller case studies, the diet has improved conditions of type 2 diabetes mellitus, autism, migraine headaches, depression, and polycystic ovary syndrome.

Furthermore, unregulated clinical tests showed evidences that the LCHF diet provide modifications in the activity of disease symptoms in a wider scope of neurodegenerative problems, such as Alzheimer's disease, amyotrophic lateral sclerosis, and Parkinson's disease.

Whereas, the brain's glucose metabolism is impaired in Alzheimer's disease, neurological studies invoke suggestions that ketone bodies may offer an alternative energy source for the brain. Thus, the LCHF diet may also be a protective mechanism in strokes and traumatic brain injuries. Since tumor cells are ineffective to burn ketones for energy, the LCHF diet is also recommendable as a treatment for cancer, like glioma brain tumor.

Although a 2013 medical review stated that, LCHF diets provided sufficient suggestions of possible benefits to cancer therapy, the only proof of benefit at present is anecdotal. Nevertheless, devising effective tests to measure the effects of applying a LCHF diet in cancer treatment can be challenging.

Chapter 8 – Program's Practice Pointers

Tips and Techniques

While it is not necessary monitoring your daily intake of carbohydrates and calories, it definitely helps knowing exactly what you are consuming in order for you to point out easily missteps along the way. It would be more beneficial to learn a few tips towards your success in engaging with the LCHF diet:

1. Avoid processed and canned foods if you can. Obviously, you are always unsure of their origins, derivations, and compositions, not to mention their unhealthy and diminished nutritional values.

2. Always remember the recommended and appropriate items for each food group. In this way, it facilitates you knowing what foods are necessary for consumption and those to avoid.

3. Know your macros or macronutrient consumptions. These consumptions

include the three major nutrients—protein, fats, and net carbohydrate intake. Net carb consumption is your total dietary carbohydrates less your total fiber intakes. Being aware of your macros allows you to gauge the quantities of calories you need to consume, together with the proteins, fats, and carbohydrates in order to meeting your goals and achieving a successful LCHF diet.

4. Be aware of your activity levels. It provides you with a more realistic perspective at the average quantities of calories, which your body requires to burn daily.

5. Be selective with your goals and only always apply a10 to 15%calorie surplus ora 20 to 25%calorie deficit. Based upon studies, exceeding such deficit values may incur negative impacts regarding your dieting.

6. While the LCHF diet is a great way to build up muscles, you must understand that protein intake is the key and

responsible for growing muscles and strengthening tissues. Thus, if you are planning to gain muscular mass, you must consume about 1.0 to 1.2gof protein per lean pound of your body weight.

7. The LCHF diet is not associated with a high fat consumption that causes various health problems. Rather, it is a high fat and high carbohydrates intake, which is always the culprit. Nevertheless, always consult with your physician about your concerns of the LCHF diet.

8. About sugar cravings, medical studies have evidences connecting them to artificial sweeteners. So, when using hefty amounts of artificial sweeteners or drinkingdiet sodas, try skipping them altogether and modify your eating habits, lifestyles and philosophies.

9. There is truly no real harm involving yourself with the LCHF diet lest you have a history of health issues concerning your kidney or acquiring

Type-1 diabetes. Only ensure knowing that the first few days along the diet usually provide you some severe headaches and lethargic moods and movements as your body begins to adapt to the discipline. Allow a few weeks to get the hang of it, especially its initial hump, and certainly, you will curb your usual cravings for carbohydrates.

10. It has been a common misconception that the LCHF diet seems to be expensive. Upon seeing a low-carbohydrate diet, people will be thinking and estimating the high costs of meat. Fortunately, this is an erroneous perspective since the LCHF diet focuses moderately on protein and more on fats, which allows more savings by emphasizing primarily on the fats.

11. Once focused starting on a healthier and more realistic approach of losing body fat, indulging in a low carbohydrate diet and lifestyle is

worthwhile. The key to success concerning any diet is preparing your food in advance, or, simply creating a meal plan. A definite guideline keeps you focused and not veering away from your objectives, as well as the purposes of the diet itself.

12. While wanting to keep your carbohydrates restricted, your inclination of food consumption must principally come fromdairy, nuts, and vegetables.Most of your meals must comprise proteins with vegetables, including ample amounts of fats.

13. When you find yourself famished throughout your day, try curbing your appetite by snacking out on peanut butter, cheeses, seeds, and nuts. Snacks are also part of your meal plan, and ought to be under regulation.

14. Getting quickly into a state of ketosis depends upon your food consumption. You must be restrictive on your carbohydrates consumption, which only allows you less than 15g daily.

15. To maximize your results under the LCHF diet, achieve undergoing optimal ketosis. However, this is not recommendable for individuals suffering from Type-1 diabetes. The trick here is to not only restrict you from partaking carbohydrates, but also be aware of your protein intake. The secret, unbelievably, is having your fill with lots of fats!

Dining-out Do's & Don'ts

It always happens to the best of us when we have to drop by a fast food outlet or a fancied restaurant! We sometimes have no time cooking our food as we get into some tight schedules like staying late for overtime work, being busy hour after hour, becoming mobile on the road; or perhaps, getting into some other circumstances like, an out of town trip or attending parties that do not allow us preparing our own food.

As such, there will be tendencies that knock you out of the LCHF diet and possibilities of eating foods, which you deem as right within the bounds of the dietary program, but unknowing and clueless that carbohydrates are sneakily hiding in your food's composition.

Worry not, as you can still be able to stick to your low-carbohydrate meal plan and stay on course along your dietary program by following the options and handy tips below. These may somehow help you out, making the best choice for your situation.

- It is always primordial to bear in mind to cut out on your carbohydrates. So, know the contents and values of your food.

- Prefer salads and selected fruits as your alternatives for carbohydrates.

- Always ask to verify whether served food has traces of sugar; better still, ask and check its composition prior to ordering.

- Ensure that you are not reading a menu from a soy-based vegetarian restaurant.

- Opt for places that may feed you substantially with meat or seafood; yet, be aware about their derivation, whether or not meat comes from grain or corn-fed cows or seafood fed with soy.

- When at a fast food diner, take the buns off the doggie or burger. Better, request wrapping your burger in fresh lettuce leaves, and eat it using a fork.

- Beware of noodles and pastas derived from whole-wheat grains.

- Ask olive oil or melted butter to attain or retain your LCHF diet ratios.

- Be careful with dressings and sauces. They may contain lots of sugar. Prefer fast food chains offering salads with low-carbohydrate dressings.

- Opt for roasted, grilled, or broiled chicken over breaded or battered. When you have no options, you may peel off the skin, taking off its carbohydrates.

- When hitting the road and finding yourself hungry midst a gas station, choose filling out your tummy with deli meat, string cheese, and hard-boiled eggs, in addition to other permissible snack items such as pork rinds and almonds.

With coffee, order an Americano, which is an espresso blended in hot water; or, a Depth Charge, also known as Turbo, Sling Blade, Shot In The Dark, and Red Eye, which is a shot of espresso blended to another drip coffee brew; in short, a double espresso. Include requesting unsweetened heavy whipping cream, coconut milk, and almonds.

Conclusion

LCHF diets relatively emphasize the composition of foods that are rich in natural fats and sufficient in protein, while restricting foods that are high in carbohydrates.

While the standard American diet (SAD) comprises about 45-65% of calories taken from carbohydrates, LCHF diets limit carbohydrate consumption to only 2-4% of calories.

It is noteworthy that the low-carb high-fat diet is not a high-protein regimen, contrary to what many people and pseudo-experts think. It is actually a high-fat diet with moderated and regulated protein consumption, and a greatly reduced carbohydrate allowance. A typical LCHF meal generally consists of small quantities of protein, a source of natural or organic fats and some green leafy vegetables.

The working principle behind the diet is using ketones as a substitute energy source. When digesting foods containing carbohydrates, they are metabolically broken down into glucose in the body. With larger carbohydrate consumptions, blood sugar levels increase, or an occurrence of more glucose.

Diabetics understand that a high blood sugar is dangerous to the body. Consuming more fats and protein and less carbohydrates leads to a shift in our body metabolism, which taps to use our stored fats to convert them into energy in lieu of burning sugar or glucose. The shift produces more ketone bodies, and at the same time, decreases blood sugar levels.

When glucose drops and ketone bodies rise and dominate in the bloodstream, the heart, muscle, brain and other body organs cease to burn sugar. Rather, they use the ketone bodies as an alternative fuel source and nutritional or optimal ketosis is established.

Soon as the body applies ketones as major fuel sources, a wide variety of beneficial effects ensue. A ketone-producing, high fat, low-carb diet is truly great for reducing weight, slowing the aging process and addressing a wide array of health issues.

In fact, LCHF diets are greatly more powerful than the more popular and trendy regimen would suggest. Both anti-inflammatory and anti-oxidant effects of nutritional ketosis prove to be potent. Currently, medical research and studies still continue to explore more about nutritional or optimal ketosis for further applications and benefits it may bestow to humankind.

Overall, eating a high amount of fat, moderate protein, and low amount of carbohydrates can have a massive impact in your health— lowering your body weight, cholesterol and blood sugar, while raising your energy and mood levels. Indeed, being under the state of ketosis can certainly alleviate and augment in the treatment of several serious health issues.

As a summary, the LCHF diet is neither a trend nor a current fad. It is a powerful regulator of metabolic disorders. When implemented properly, it is capable of being extremely effective. The bottom line for LCHF diets is how you can enhance or increase your energy levels, get fit and trim, and improve your health by simply altering the way you eat.

Part 2

Chapter One

What to Eat for Breakfast While Trying to Lose Weight

Breakfast is the most important meal of the day. The reason is, because we must have something in our bodies to burn calories off in the beginning of the day. If we don't have any substances in our stomachs, then there will be nothing to give us energy or food to burn throughout the day.

Eating a healthy breakfast will give you the power to concentrate better in the mornings and will all around put you in a good mood in the very beginning of the day. It is known that people who eat breakfast every morning are more fit than those who skip it.

In this chapter, you will find different types of food to eat for breakfast while on a low-carb diet.

Eggs

Eggs are a great protein to start out the day. Starting with a traditional breakfast, only eat two eggs in the morning. Try not to exceed eating more eggs than that. Eggs are known to keep your stomach fuller as opposed to eating any other type of food for breakfast. A nice healthy side with eggs as opposed to toast; sauteed fresh spinach with a little salt and pepper to eat with your eggs in the morning.

Another great and quick breakfast: Get a whole wheat pita, scramble egg whites, add spinach, and add tomatoes for a nice healthy breakfast sandwich.

To be sure you have enough time to eat breakfast in the mornings before going to work, boil eggs the night before and place them in the refrigerator. The next morning on your way out of the door, grab two boiled eggs, you may put a little salt or pepper on them for flavor to eat on your way to work. I know how hard it is to wake up earlier than you have to, so this is a great way to be sure you aren't grabbing a bagel on your way out of the house for a quick unhealthy breakfast.

Fruit

All of these fruits listed below are full of minerals and vitamins, which our bodies need to function properly and to be healthy.

- Apples
- Bananas
- Blueberries
- Strawberries
- Raspberries
- Peach's
- Grapes
- Pineapples
- Cranberries
- Orange's
- Grapefruit
- Kiwi
- Cantaloupe
- Blackberries
- Watermelon

In the morning for a nice healthy light breakfast, cut up bananas and apples, mix them together in a bowl with blueberries and grapes. There isn't much to this, so you could eat it just by itself or if you would like, eat this as a side with eggs.

Peach's are great with a little cottage cheese and almonds mixed together for a nice light breakfast.

There are many different types of fruit which are good in oatmeal, but my personal favorite is to mix a little bit of almond milk with bananas and blueberries into my oatmeal in the mornings.

There are many different types of oats, which are great if mixed with a little honey, almond milk, and your choice of fruit or raisins.

Another great breakfast with any of these fruits, would be making a breakfast smoothie blended with plain Greek yogurt and honey.

Take apple slices and dip them into peanut butter in the mornings. The fiber from the peanut butter will help keep you full up until lunch time.

Plain Greek yogurt is a nice creamy breakfast add honey as a sweetener and your choice of different types of fruit and nuts to mix into the yogurt.

Grapefruit is a wonderful fruit to eat when trying to lose weight. It is best to eat half of a grapefruit before eating breakfast in the mornings. Don't just eat grapefruit by itself. This would be a great fruit to pair with a protein, such as eggs or Greek yogurt.

Almond butter is delicious and healthy. A great way to eat it in the mornings is to spread it onto bananas or apples.

Chopped watermelon and cantaloupe are a great side to eat with any breakfast. These two fruits are very good for your health and they are a nice sweet snack to go along with a well rounded healthy breakfast.

Protein

There are many different types of protein to add to your breakfast in the mornings other than eggs and yogurt, here is a list of other types of healthy protein breakfast ideas:

Spread low fat cottage cheese onto a whole wheat piece of toast.

Instead of putting bacon, sausage, or ham into an omelet, put diced pieces of chicken instead.

Instead of making scrambled eggs, make scrambled tofu. Add mushrooms, spinach, tomatoes, broccoli, onions, peppers, or any other vegetable of your liking low in carbohydrates to the tofu breakfast scramble.

Wrap turkey bacon around pieces of avocados and place them in the oven for about five minutes on 350 degrees.

Toast whole wheat bread, spread apple butter or peanut butter on the toast, and add sliced bananas on top.

Heat up quinoa in the microwave as a substitute for oatmeal, add cinnamon, sliced apples or blueberries, and mix in a few almonds or walnuts.

Make a protein shake in the morning with your favorite type of protein powder. This is very filling and it is easy and very quick to make. I like to mix two scoops of vanilla protein into one cup of soy milk.

Chapter Two

Different Types of Food for Lunch to Help you Lose Weight

Breakfast is not the only important meal of the day. Making sure you eat a healthy low-carb lunch is very important to keep your high energy flowing throughout the entire day.

It is extremely important while on a diet to not skip any meals, as our bodies need the substances to burn off calories to help us lose weight.

In this chapter you will be learning about different lunch ideas to help you lose weight, while on a low-carb diet.

Salads

A salad made up of different types of lettuce such as: arugula, romaine lettuce, butter lettuce, and watercress are all full of nutrition. Try to stay away from eating only iceberg lettuce, because it doesn't have much nutritional value to it. Here is a list of different types of salads to eat for lunch while trying to lose weight:

Kale and salmon Caesar salad. Only mix about a teaspoon full of light Caesar dressing onto the kale. Instead of salmon, you could also use grilled chicken, sauteed shrimp, or white fish.

Romaine lettuce mixed with fresh spinach. Add vegetables to your liking such as: tomatoes, cucumbers, olives, green beans, avocados, and yellow or green bell peppers. For protein add diced turkey, diced chicken, or shrimp. For a light homemade dressing: Squeeze a quarter of a lemon into a bowl, mix in garlic powder, white wine vinegar, a touch of salt, and a pinch of pepper.

Sliced tomatoes with mozzarella cheese and basil. Drizzle a very light balsamic dressing and olive oil on top.

Arugula, butter lettuce, and watercress lettuce mixed with tomatoes, cabbage, goat cheese, cucumbers, red onions, with a light vinaigrette and oil for dressing. Add your choice of protein: flank steak, diced chicken, fish, or shrimp.

More lunch items to eat while trying to lose weight:

Lettuce wraps- Make chicken on the stove, add ginger, soy sauce, and garlic. Take shredded carrots and diced cucumbers to add on top with a garnish of a few sesame seeds. This wrap would taste wonderful with either a butter lettuce leaf or cabbage leaf.

Tortilla wraps- Take deli turkey or deli chicken and wrap it into a whole wheat tortilla. Add romaine lettuce, tomatoes, onions, and a little bit of olive oil and red wine vinegar for flavor.

Burrito- Make a bean burrito with re-fried or black beans, guacamole, and salsa. Instead of using a tortilla, mix everything in a bowl. Add fresh tomatoes or lettuce if you would like. As a side to eat with this burrito instead of rice, have a cup of fresh fruit.

Tuna salad- Mix tuna with chopped celery, chopped onion, pepper, a pinch of salt, and a teaspoon of lemon juice. Slice a tomato and chop lettuce to add to the tuna salad.

Quinoa- Make quinoa on the stove. After it is cooked you may eat this cold or hot; to your liking. For more flavor and nutrition add chopped tomatoes, chopped chives or onions, cucumber, and fresh herbs- basil, cilantro, oregano, or thyme.

Chop a whole head of cauliflower, mix it with a little olive oil, and add your choice of seasonings. Set the oven on broil and cook the cauliflower on low for ten minutes. At the same time cook the quinoa on the stove for about 15 minutes. Cook kale separately on the stove. After they are all done cooking, mix the cauliflower, quinoa, and kale together for a light lunch.

Turkey burger- Make a turkey burger on the stove, grill, or in the oven. Instead of eating it with a bun, get some fresh spinach, tomatoes, onions, and a dab of ketchup or mustard for flavor.

Soup- This is a low-calorie meal depending on what kind of homemade soup you make. Buy bags of frozen vegetables from the grocery store as well as fresh vegetables. Use low-sodium chicken broth for a base as well as water. For protein add chicken or beans. For flavor add garlic and fresh herbs. The best way to make this: Put all of the ingredients in a crock pot and cook on low for six hours. Add your favorite seasonings and herbs for more flavor.

Cottage Cheese- Make a mix of cottage cheese, grapes, avocados, cucumbers, and tomatoes. Add cracked pepper on top.

Healthy Sandwich- Make a sandwich without the bread by slicing cucumbers, deli turkey, a little cheese, and put them together by using a toothpick to hold them in place.

Stir Fry- Chopped chicken with broccoli, red and green bell peppers, squash, and red onions. Use olive oil and a low-sodium teriyaki sauce to cook these ingredients up on the stove on medium-high heat for ten minutes.

Avocado Salad- Slice an avocado in half, take the pit out from the center and add in homemade low fat chicken salad or tuna salad to the middle of the avocado.

Hummus Wrap- Make a whole wheat wrap with hummus, goat cheese, turkey slices, and fresh spinach leaves.

Quinoa Wrap- Make a quinoa wrap with black beans, feta cheese, and avocado rolled all together in a whole wheat wrap. Add humus for flavor.

As a side with any of these entrees, it is a good idea to mix them together. For instance; making a salad and having a cup of soup as the side or with the wraps have a side of fruit or vegetables.

Chapter Three

A List of Snacks While Trying to Lose weight

Snacking on different types of healthy foods throughout the day helps our bodies get all of the good nutrition that we need. It is known that if we eat every three to four hours our blood sugar will stay steady and we will feel a lot more energized throughout the entire day. Try to stick to snack foods which will help you burn fat, but don't over indulge. Stay away from snacks such as chips or cookies.

A great idea to make sure you have snacks ready to go when walking out the door, put them all in Tupperware or Ziploc bags in the refrigerator or in the kitchen cabinet. This way you can just grab them and they are already packaged up with the right amount of food.

Here is a list of different types of healthy snacks to eat while on a diet:

Fruit is a great food to snack on. There are many different types of fruit which could be easy to grab and they are all full of vitamins and minerals, which our bodies need everyday.

Chopping up different types of vegetables such as; cucumbers, carrots, celery, peppers, olives, broccoli, or cauliflower and dip them into hummus.

Cottage cheese with peaches or cantaloupe.

Goat cheese spread on top of sliced tomatoes.

Apples or celery with peanut butter.

Deli turkey rolled up with low fat cheese.

Freeze bananas and pieces of mango. Mix them together for a sweet slushie snack.

Make your own homemade butter-free popcorn, by substituting a little olive oil. Add a tiny amount of salt for taste.

Boil shrimp and then chill it. Make your very own homemade cocktail sauce with horseradish, lemon juice, cracked pepper, and a tiny bit of ketchup for dipping.

Make a mix of raisins, dried cranberries, cashews, walnuts, pecans, and almonds. Put them in Ziploc bags, so they are ready to go.

Make homemade guacamole. Cut up a stalk of celery and dip the celery pieces into the guacamole.

You can buy frozen edamame in the grocery store. Heat it up in the microwave, and add a little salt to it.

Nuts are always a great snack to eat while on a diet. Pistachios and almonds are known to be less fattening as compared to other nuts and they are very filling. Try not to exceed more than 20 nuts in one sitting.

Heat up a whole artichoke in the microwave. Separately heat up olive oil with salt, garlic, and pepper to dip the artichoke hearts into.

Sugar-free applesauce. If you like cinnamon, sprinkle a dash into the applesauce.

Make your own vegetable dip with plain Greek low-fat yogurt, onion powder, celery salt, and garlic powder. Add salt and pepper to your liking.

Vegetables for the homemade dip: carrots, celery, red or green bell peppers, cucumbers, tomatoes, broccoli, or cauliflower.

Pizza bites made with sliced eggplant, tomato sauce, with a very small amount of feta and mozzarella cheese on top. Put all of the ingredients together and bake in the oven.

Deli ham slices wrapped with sliced apples and low-fat cheese.

Sliced cucumbers with light cream cheese spread on top. (Do not use more than one tablespoon of cream cheese).

Chopped red peppers with goat cheese for dipping. (Do not use more than one tablespoon of goat cheese).

Cut slices of kiwi and sprinkle shredded coconut on top.

And last, but not least, one of my favorite snacks: Frozen red grapes.

Chapter Four

Different Types of Food to Eat For Dinner While on a Diet

Dinner is the last meal of the day, so make sure you do not eat too close to bedtime, because our bodies need time to burn the calories off. To make sure you are eating healthy, have a set dinner plan for each night of the week. That way you can pull whatever meat is in the freezer to defrost in the refrigerator during the day.

In this chapter, there will be a list of different types of food to eat for dinner to help you lose weight while on a low-carb diet.

Chicken

Making boneless-skinless chicken breasts on the grill with very light olive oil and topped with seasonings (my favorite seasoning on chicken is a Greek seasoning called Cavender's). For sides; cut zucchini in long strips, sliced mushrooms, and asparagus. Wrap these vegetables in aluminum foil and coat them with a little olive oil and your choice of seasonings for flavor. And place these directly onto the grill.

Bake chicken in the oven topped with lemon juice and rosemary. For sides boil red skinned potatoes and roasted kale.

Make a chicken Caesar salad with kale and romaine lettuce, mix in a teaspoon of light Caesar dressing, and add grilled or baked chicken. Add a dash of Parmesan cheese on top.

Bake chicken in the oven with lemon juice, spices, and capers. Add basil or cilantro for flavor. As a side make Brussels sprouts in the oven on bake for about ten minutes and the last remaining two minutes set the oven to broil on high so they are a little crispy. Brush the Brussels sprouts with a little olive oil and add your choice of seasonings for flavor before putting them into the oven.

Sauteed chicken with ginger and garlic on the stove. Separately sauteed spinach, mushrooms, and onions. Lay the vegetables down first on the plate and top them with chicken and sprinkle sesame seeds onto the dish.

A great healthy, homemade, chicken and vegetable crock pot soup dinner- Put water on the bottom, add a whole chicken, cut up carrots, celery, and bok choy or kale. Add a bag of mixed frozen vegetables. Add garlic powder, chopped parsley, pepper, and a dash of salt. Make sure to shred the chicken and dispose of the carcass when it is done cooking. Cook all of the ingredients on low for six hours.

Sauteed bean sprouts and diced green bell peppers with olive oil, red pepper flakes, garlic, and a little soy sauce. Separately, sauteed diced chicken with ginger and garlic. Once the chicken is fully cooked, go ahead and mix the vegetables and chicken together.

Seafood

Shrimp sauteed with fresh spinach, chopped zucchini, chopped broccoli, chopped carrots and cauliflower. Cook this all on the stove with fresh herbs and seasonings to your liking. Only cook this with olive oil. Do not use any butter.

Bake salmon in the oven with capers, lemon juice, and olive oil. For a side with the salmon, steam broccoli or asparagus.

Cook shrimp on the stove with garlic, pepper, lemon juice, a dash of salt, and chicken broth. Boil whole wheat pasta on the stove. Chop kalamata olives, onions, cilantro, and tomatoes to add to the pasta. Mix all of the ingredients together including the sauce left over, which the shrimp was cooked in.

Wrap salmon in foil and add tomatoes, onions, garlic, capers, and lemon juice on top of the salmon. Wrap all of the ingredients up and put them in the oven and bake at 350 degrees for twenty minutes.

Grill or sear white fish with lemon juice, capers, cilantro, and garlic. Make a green vegetable as a side; such as kale, broccoli, asparagus, or spinach.

Pork

Boneless pork chops made on the stove with white or red cooking wine with spices. Separately cook mushrooms on the stove with olive oil, minced garlic, salt, and pepper. Make fresh steamed greens beans. Pour the mushrooms over the pork chops and eat the green beans as a side.

Grill pork chops and slices of pineapple. For a nice flavor, marinade the pork with a low-sodium soy sauce, ginger, and garlic. For a side make brown rice on the stove with chopped red and green bell peppers.

Pork tacos. Make the pork in the crock pot with a light barbeque seasoning. Chop onions, cilantro, tomatoes, and mangoes for toppings. For flavor add guacamole to a whole wheat soft taco shell with the rest of the ingredients. Squeeze fresh lime juice on top for extra flavor.

Other healthy dinners

For a taco salad; cook ground turkey on the stove. Chop tomatoes, cilantro, and onions. For the lettuce use romaine lettuce. If you would like to add cheese, use a fat-free shredded cheddar cheese. For dressing add a little salsa and guacamole. As a side make brown rice and black beans.

Grill steak with peppercorn seasoning on top. Mix tomatoes, onions, cucumbers, sprouts, feta cheese, romaine lettuce, and cabbage in a light oil and vinegar based dressing and add the peppercorn grilled steak on top.

For another nice dinner salad; grill flank steak, chop avocados, tomatoes, cucumbers, add a dab of goat cheese, arugula, and romaine lettuce. For dressing use oil and vinegar or your own homemade dressing with lemon juice, white wine vinegar, garlic powder, and a touch of salt and pepper.

Make a large plate of grilled vegetables. Such as: zucchini, eggplant, onions, tomatoes, carrots, peppers, portobello mushrooms, and Brussels sprouts. Brush all of the vegetables with a light coat of olive oil with a little salt and pepper.

Multi-grain pasta mixed with fresh vegetables. Cook the pasta separately. And saute the vegetables in a pan with a tablespoon of olive oil. When they are all done cooking, mix the vegetables and pasta with a basil pesto or tomato sauce.

Vegetables: asparagus, mushrooms, spinach, squash, and tomatoes.

Weight Loss Journey Conclusion

I hope this is a good starting guide on what to eat to help you lose weight. While on a diet, it is a good idea to keep up with morning and nightly exercises to get the best results during and after your low-carb diet. Try not to eat many carbohydrates or sweets. Make sure you are making goals every week and try your best to stick to them.

Dieting is an extremely hard task, but with the right mindset and the willpower to do it, it can be done. Make sure you are setting time aside to work out. Every morning try and wake up a little earlier than usual and just do a light jog before work. Before going to bed, wait about thirty minutes after eating dinner and do the same thing again. If you have a gym membership head over to the gym before and after work.

Make sure when going on a diet, if you are married to get your spouse on board, as well. It will make your weight loss journey so much easier when you both are dieting at the same time. This way you will be not tempted to eat certain foods or skip out on exercising. Do it together as a team.

Make sure to take lunch with you every day to work, this way you will not be tempted to buy something unhealthy or unsatisfying. Be sure to have a meal plan set out for every evening, so when you get home it's all right there ready to cook, this way you won't be tempted to order a pizza or another type of fast food.

Stay strong while going on a low-carb diet. Keep reminding yourself what your goals are when you start to think about ice cream, chips, cookies, etc... There was a reason why you started this diet, you will have so much more energy after eating healthy just after three days. Try not to weigh yourself every day. Only weigh yourself once a week and write down in a journal each week what your weight is, so you can see how far you have come.

Conclusion

It is my sincere hope that you might have liked all the recipes which have been mentioned in the book and once again thank you for getting this book and experimenting with the recipes.

About The Author

Norman Wheeler is born with the vision to promote the art of *Low Carb* cooking among the masses. The author has written several research papers on the topic. He has served as an instructor promoting various cultural arts in University of San Francisco. He is currently living with his spouse in Texas.

www.ingramcontent.com/pod-product-compliance
Lightning Source LLC
LaVergne TN
LVHW011945070526
838202LV00054B/4807